# CRITICAL THINKING ACTIVITIES for NURSING

# CRITICAL THINKING ACTIVITIES for NURSING

**Marilyn Smith-Stoner,** RN, MSN

Faculty Member
University of Phoenix
Ontario, California

Doctoral Student
California Institute of Integral Studies
San Francisco, California

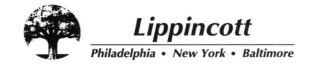
**Lippincott**
Philadelphia • New York • Baltimore

*Acquisitions Editor: Susan Keneally*
*Production Editor: Jahmae Harris*
*Senior Production Manager: Helen Ewan*
*Senior Production Coordinator: Nannette Winski*
*Assistant Art Director: Kathy Kelley-Luedtke*
*Printer: Victor Graphics, Inc.*
*Compositor: Pine Tree Composition, Inc.*

**Library of Congress Cataloging in Publication Data**

Smith-Stoner, Marilyn.
    Critical thinking activities for nursing / Marilyn Smith-Stoner.
       p.     cm.
    Includes bibliographical references and index.
    ISBN 0–7817–1619–5
    1. Nursing—Philosophy.  2. Critical thinking.  I. Title.
    [DNLM:  1. Nursing Process.  2. Problem-Based Learning nurses'
instruction.  3. Thinking nurses' instruction.  WY  100  S661c  1998]
    RT84.5.S575  1998
    610.73—dc21
    DNLM/DLC
    for Library of Congress                98–3973
                                         CIP

9    8    7    6    5    4    3    2    1

CRITICALTHINKINGCRITICALTHINKINGCRITICALTHINKINGCRITICALTHINKINGCRITICAL
THINKINGCRITICALTHINKINGCRITICALTHINKINGCRITICALTHINKINGCRITICALTHINKING
CRITICALTHINKINGCRITICALTHINKINGCRITICALTHINKINGCRITICALTHINKINGCRITICAL
THINKINGCRITICALTHINKINGCRITICALTHINKINGCRITICALTHINKINGCRITICALTHINKING
CRITICALTHINKINGCRITICALTHINKINGCRITICALTHINKINGCRITICALTHINKINGCRITICAL

# DEDICATION

I dedicate the following poem written by an unknown author for the many nursing students who will use this book. It is different from other texts. It invites you to become part of the book. It may be scary to have to think on your own. We do not educate students to think creatively in this country. Few courses and even fewer role models exist to show the way to developing critical thinking skills, which are so necessary for health care workers of today and tomorrow. Your efforts will pay off! In the meantime . . .

## Don't Quit

When things go wrong, as they sometimes will,
When the road you're trudgin up seems all uphill,
When the funds are low and the doubts high,
And you want to smile, but you have to sigh,
When care is pressing you down a bit,
Rest if you must—but don't you quit.

Life is queer with its twists and turns,
The road you're trudgin up seems all uphill,
When the funds are low and the doubts high,
And you want to smile, but you have to sigh,
When care is pressing you down a bit,
Rest if you must—but don't you quit.

Often the goal is nearer than
It seems the road you're trudgin upall uphill,
When the funds are low and the doubts high,
And you want to smile, but you have to sigh,
When care is pressing you down a bit,
Rest if you must—but don't you quit.

Success is failure turned inside out—
When the road you're trudgin up seems all uphill,
When the funds are low and the doubts high,
And you want to smile, but you have to sigh,
When care is pressing you down a bit,
It's when things seem worst that you mustn't quit.

This text is dedicated also to Marlys Mayfield, my critical thinking inspiration.

# INTRODUCTION

Critical thinking is an evolving field of inquiry. There are many definitions of critical thinking in general, and in specific displines such as nursing. Whatever else critical thinking is, it involves many skills. The most significant include the synthesis of information, the ability to analyze information from many sources, and then to articulate the issues presented clearly and concisely.

## Definitions of Critical Thinking

Richard Paul, one of the country's leading experts in critical thinking defines it as:

> "The art of thinking about your thinking while you are thinking in order to make your thinking better: more clear, more accurate, or more defensible" (Paul, 1992, p. 263).

Ruest (1993, p. 56–57) defines critical thinking in nursing in the following way:

> "Critical thinking in baccalaureate nursing education is the collection, organizing, and synthesizing of information in professional situations which guide nursing actions. The thinking requires understanding abstract ideas, consideration of the context in which a situation exists, and openness to new ideas. Nursing process often provides the framework in which critical thinking occurs."

A common critical thinking definition put forth from the 1990 Delphi report from the American Psychological Association is:

> "We understand critical thinking to be purposeful, self-regulated judgement which results in interpretation, analysis, evaluation, and inference, as well as explanation of the evidential, conceptual, methodological, criteriological, or contextual considerations upon which that judgement is based. . . ."

Everyone is calling for critical thinking to be included in nursing education. But how to do it? Critical think is difficult! Henry Ford said, "Thinking is hard work, that is why so few people do it". Once critical thinking activities are identified, how can they be made interesting, even inviting? These are not easy to do. However, this book attempts to do just that.

## Benefits of Critical Thinking

Critical thinking can be challenging AND fun! It is worth the effort! I invite the reader to use this book with the attitude of an explorer. What are you exploring? Yourself! Critical thinkers first begin by examining their own ideas about the world. As you reveal more and more of your previously unexamined thought patterns, the synthesis, integration and evaluation of information gets easier. It takes work—but you will be pleased with the results.

## How is Critical Thinking Different From Problem Solving?

Problem solving is often confused with critical thinking. However, there are some important differences. Problem solving often calls for the individual to identify one, and only one, possible right answer. In critical thinking, the individual often is challenged to come up with several alternatives, which may be unique to the situation. For example, when a nurse is trying to make a patient care decision, there are professional guidelines and standards of practice which dictate many of the actions a nurse performs. Most of the actions are the only right answer, such as when to call a physician over a patient's condition or when to give a medication from a listing of standing orders.

In critical thinking, the nurse may be called on to identify a solution for a problem that has not existed before and there is no set standard of action. This book is full of real life examples of those very kinds of problems. Solutions come partly from nursing knowledge, but also from the nurse's ability to think abstractly and creatively. That is what this book is all about. Challenging yourself to think creatively—for yourself!

## What You Can Expect from This Book

You can expect to be challenged. You can expect to have to think for yourself. You can expect to have to spend time on the assignments. Most of all you can expect to learn something about yourself and how to solve complex problems in the field of nursing. Enjoy your explorations!

# CONTENTS

## CHAPTER 3
## Critical Thinking Activities Related to Death and Dying    71

## CHAPTER 4
## Critical Thinking Activities Related to Nursing Ethics    99

## CHAPTER 5
## Advanced Critical Thinking Activities    125

## CHAPTER 6
## Debate Topics    151

## APPENDIX Internet Addresses    177

# CHAPTER

# 1

# BEGINNING CRITICAL THINKING ACTIVITIES

# When Did You First Realize That You Were Going to Be a Nurse?

This may be the most important critical thinking exercise you will ever do. As a nursing student you are becoming educated and socialized into the role of a nurse as it is understood by your college or university at the present time. A considerable amount of what you have learned may have been a surprise to you and perhaps did not fit your image of what a nurse did.

There was a time when you thought you knew what a nurse did and that's what you wanted to do. That's when you decided to become a nurse. It may have been a few months to a few years before you actually started the nursing program. This image of what a nurse was like and the kind of work he or she did greatly impacted your decision to become a nurse. Now that you *know* what a nurse does, how does your image of reality match what you *thought* a nurse did?

This is an exercise to help you get back in touch with your earliest vision of nursing and determine what your underlying assumptions about your role as a nurse included.

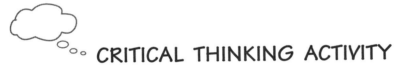 CRITICAL THINKING ACTIVITY

**Describe what you thought nursing would be when you first decided to become a nurse.** Be very specific. Consider everything about your vision and write it down. Include your total image of nursing.

Sit back and relax in a comfortable chair. Play some relaxing music if you prefer. In your mind's eye, picture yourself talking about becoming a nurse. As each image comes into your mind, try to see the one *before* the one you are seeing. You may need to do this over several sessions, especially if you have not thought about these ideas for a while. Your mind will "give up" these memories if you give it time and space to do so.

Perhaps your first image of what a nurse is came from a book or a television show. Maybe your were ill and had direct contact with nurses. Is there a nurse in your family or church who influenced you? Did you see a salary survey and realize that nurses were paid an acceptable wage, compared with others?

What kind of work did you picture yourself doing? What kind of patients were you taking care of? Where did you work? What was your relationship to the physicians and other nurses you worked with? Did you see any difficulties or problems with nursing? Or was your image one of occupational serenity and satisfaction?

Did you think you would have friends who were nurses? Who would your spouse be—a nurse or other health care worker?

What did you think would happen in a regular shift? What specific types of jobs would you be doing? You may want to draw yourself as a nurse to help you get started.

**Compare and contrast your original image of nursing with the one you hold today.** Is it possible to keep both your dream of what you wanted a nurse to be and your knowledge of what a nurse is? If so, why? If not, why not?

# Create Your Own Holiday

Just about any subject can be celebrated. Many events we take for granted are potential subjects for celebration. Consider the following list of possibly unlikely party themes.

Handwriting Analysis Week

National Clean Off Your Desk Week

International Thank-You Day

Clean Out Your Computer Day

American Chocolate Week

National Anxiety Month

Bird Day

Rubber Eraser Day

National Third Shift Worker Day

Save the Rhino Day

National Forgiveness Day

International Left Handers Day

Petroleum Day

National Be Late For Something Day

Dictionary Day

National Magic Day

Sinkie Day (the day you eat over a sink)

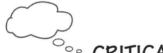 CRITICAL THINKING ACTIVITY

Have you ever celebrated one of these holidays? **Think about what goes into a holiday or ritual celebration.** What events do people celebrate? What happens during the event to keep people wanting to repeat the celebration? How do the new people become acquainted with the celebration? Is participation restricted based on race, gender, age, or some other characteristic? How does the same holiday vary from culture to culture and throughout time? How do social institutions like organized religion impact the celebration of various holidays? How does health or illness impact celebrations? How many rituals can you identify that focus on health or healing?

Consider this: when euthanasia is legalized, who will help define the rituals related to the final act of taking a person's life? Do you think American society will develop rituals such as a birth that everyone comes to watch? Or will the rituals be more like confessing one's sins—done in private with some degree of secrecy?

Now it's your turn! **Come up with your own unique holiday after getting some inspiration from the list.** Name your holiday, describe it's purpose in detail, and explain why you think it is significant. Also describe any rituals you think should be performed to celebrate the holiday. Be as creative as you can be! Include a description of the traditional foods, activities, and other important features of your holiday. Consider setting aside a day to celebrate one of the new holidays your class creates.

# Medication Discovery

Patients have a variety of experiences related to illness and disease. Not all of their suffering can be alleviated by medication, treatments, or surgery. Some patients must endure long periods of time away from family and friends. Some lose a limb; others endure loss of senses such as sight or hearing. Fear of disability and death are also problems, among many other issues. Long-term care facilities are full of individuals who have suffered the loss of a role, or a position in a family, and disability. Rehabilitation facilities of all kinds treat patients who will never again be able to live the life they once had. Although many successfully reestablish a meaningful life for themselves, they often are left with a feeling of having lost something precious.

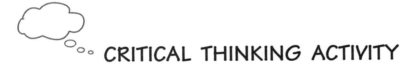 CRITICAL THINKING ACTIVITY

You have an opportunity to "discover" a medication. This is an unconventional kind of medication. It can treat any condition you feel needs a cure. It does not have to be a standard medical treatment. **What medication will you invent? What condition will it treat?**

Think about your clinical placements. How did you feel about the patients you took care of? Did you feel all of their problems were taken care of in a meaningful way? Were some things left undone or unable to be solved? Here's your chance to "fix" that problem. Identify the medication for your problem. Name it, give it a route, a dose, and a frequency and indicate which patients this medication is suitable for. How much should this medication cost? What are the side effects? What does the medication look like?

**Challenge yourself further by developing an ad to "sell" this medication.**

# HINTS HINTS HINTS HINTS HINTS

Take a walk around the halls of a health care facility. Look around and try to see what is "behind" the obvious images. What do the people coming there for treatment really need? Talk with health care workers there and see what unmet needs they feel patients have and work from there.

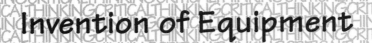

# Invention of Equipment

We are in the middle of another technological revolution in health care. Machines that can replace a human heart, liver, or pancreas are being developed and perfected all over the world. Computers are replacing paper charts. Computerized machines now store and record medication distribution. Who knows what technological breakthrough will be next?

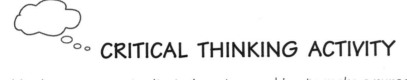

## CRITICAL THINKING ACTIVITY

You have an opportunity to invent a machine *to make a nurse's work easier*. **What piece of equipment will you invent to help nurses perform their jobs more easily?**

Select an area of the hospital, the home, or other health care facility for demonstration of this equipment. What are the challenges of patient care in that setting? What common jobs need to be automated or streamlined? What are the concerns of nurses working on that unit? What do they think is necessary to assist them to do their jobs?

This must be a unique piece of equipment not currently on the market. You also need to draw this piece of equipment and develop an owner's manual with instructions for use.

**Challenge yourself further by developing an ad to sell this piece of equipment.**

## HINTS HINTS HINTS HINTS HINTS

Take a walk around a selected unit. What are the most common jobs done by the staff? What jobs are particularly difficult? What do nurses want help with? What do you experience when you work on this unit? How can the job be simplified and made more efficient?

# Sufi Mystical Tradition

There was a farmer who had a horse, and the horse ran away. His neighbor said, ". . . too bad . . . you lost your horse." The farmer said, "You never know".

The next day the horse came back and he was leading two wild horses. His neighbor said, ". . . lucky you, now you have three horses." The farmer said, "You never know".

The next day the farmer's son was trying to tame one of the wild horses and fell off, breaking his leg. The neighbor said, ". . . too bad . . . your son can't help you anymore." The farmer said, "You never know."

The next day the army came through and took all the young men, but they didn't take the farmer's son because he had a broken leg. The neighbor said, "Lucky you, they didn't take your son." And the farmer said. . . .

 CRITICAL THINKING ACTIVITY

Read the passage through several times. Think about its obvious and deeper meanings. **Consider a situation that you initially found troubling but later reframed.** Use any method to illustrate how your change in perception occurred. Draw a diagram relating the perceptions. Use lines, dots, drawings—whatever clearly describes the process by which your perception changed.

To reframe: The process of examining an event in your life and reconstructing the meaning of this event as a result of new information, reflection on underlying assumptions, and dialogue.

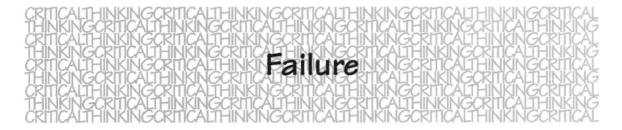

# Failure

## Lydia Maria Child, 1868

All who strive to live for something beyond mere selfish aims find their capacities for doing very inadequate to their aspirations. They do so much less than they want to do, and so much less than they, at the outset, expected to do, that their lives, viewed retrospectively, inevitably look like a failure.

## CRITICAL THINKING ACTIVITY

This passage is from Ms. Child's *Selected Letters, 1817–1880*. She had just turned sixty-six. **How do her thoughts from more than a hundred years ago resonate with you?**

# Prayer for A Difficult Patient to Nurse

O God,

I needn't tell you how difficult _____ is.

He is irritable and impatient and demanding;

Whatever I do is wrong.

He wouldn't be happy unless he had something to complain
about.

He will never admit that he is making progress and feeling
better.

Oh God, give me patience,

Never to let myself be angered and upset;

give me sympathy, always try to understand;

give me wisdom of mind,

to help him through his difficult time.

Keep me from becoming annoyed,

no matter what the provocation;

and help me always to keep on caring,

even when there seems to be no response.

Hasten his or her cure in body and in mind,

so that the day will soon come when the difficult time will
be forgotten.

And Lord Jesus, help me always to remember,

that whatever I have to bear,

it is nothing to the ingratitude and thanklessness that you
had to bear.

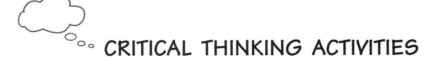

## CRITICAL THINKING ACTIVITIES

Read this prayer several times. Does it sound realistic to you? Is it possible to have a faith so deep that you can pray for patience in caring for a difficult patient and feel better? What about your faith, if you are a nonChristian? Does this prayer seem reasonable

---

From: *Prayers for Helping and Healing.* William Barclay, Augsburg, Minneapolis, MN.

from your spiritual perspective? Compose a prayer for yourself that you may use when caring for difficult patients. In your prayer, express how your faith can support the hard work of nursing. Use terms from your own spiritual tradition. Plan on sharing these prayers in small groups. Be able to describe your belief system and how prayer may positively affect your work as a nurse.

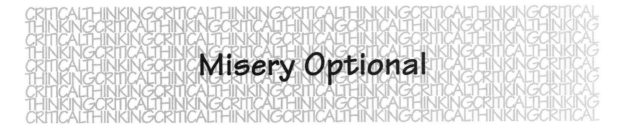

# Misery Optional

"Pain is inevitable, but misery is optional" is an often-quoted phrase in hospitals and clinics.

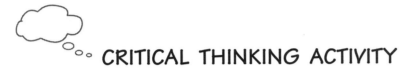

## CRITICAL THINKING ACTIVITY

Consider this phrase. Ask a few patients what they think it means. Ask your classmates what they think it means. After you have asked a number of people, from different life circumstances and ethnic backgrounds, prepare a diagram describing the similarities and differences among the meanings.

Can you identify any commonalities among the groups?

**Reflect on the meaning yourself. Define misery. Explain why misery is optional.**

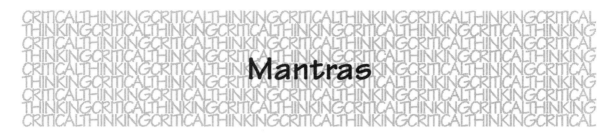

# Mantras

Mantras have been used throughout time, beginning in India many centuries ago, as a method of focusing the mind. Mantras are considered to have powerful effects on those who use them. Literally the word mantra means "the thought that liberates or protects."

Repeating a mantra can help you overcome fear, increase your creativity, give you energy when you are tired, and inspire you to keep going when you want to quit.

Many of us are very familiar with mantras but may not realize it. Our lives are filled with such mantras as "I'll never make it," or "The teacher is just out to get me," or "This is just too hard, I might as well quit now".

In some spiritual traditions, mantras are given to students by their teachers. However, it is possible to make up your own mantra and use it as an antidote to other negative mantras you may already be using.

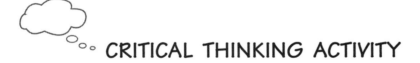

# CRITICAL THINKING ACTIVITY

**Design a mantra for your personal use in nursing school.** This mantra will be a simple phrase that you will recite over and over in times of need or when preparing for course work or patient care. Write this mantra down. Use it consciously for 2 weeks. Record the effect it has on you. Is this something you find beneficial? Describe your reactions in detail.

# HINTS HINTS HINTS HINTS HINTS

Mantras are words deliberately put together. They can be recited but are often sung to a simple melody. The words or sounds in the mantra you create should be positive and special to you. The mantra should be easy to remember and something that makes you slow down and become more mindful or aware of what you are doing.

From *Mantras: Words of Power.* Swami Sivananda Rash, Timeless Books, PO Box 3543, Spokane Washington, 99220-3543. 509-838-6652

# Nursing The Whole Family

A 68-year-old woman is being cared for at home after a stroke. She is able to get out of bed and use the bedside commode unaided, but she cannot do much more than that. Her husband and adult children care for her on a daily basis. In general they do a satisfactory job, except for the fact that they will not empty the bucket on the commode. When the home care nurse or home health aide comes for a visit, the bucket is always full and the room has the stench of feces and urine.

The case manager has been to the home and discussed this with the family on several occasions. The patient does not seem to object to the stench. The family is adamant that this is the job of the nurses. The nurse has educated the family in aesthetics, infection control, and the possible adverse effects of leaving the products of elimination in the bucket for 2 to 3 days. Nothing so far has worked.

The home health aide has also expressed her concern to the family and to the team in patient care meetings. It is getting to the point where no one wants to go to the home.

## CRITICAL THINKING ACTIVITY

You are the new home care nurse assigned to the patient. You've decided that this is a problem with a solution. **Approach the family with a new and fresh attitude toward the problem that will solve this stinky issue once and for all.** Keep in mind your legal, ethical, and personal responsibilities and limitations.

## HINTS HINTS HINTS HINTS HINTS

You may want to role play your approach with several different students. You also may want to videotape your interactions with another student and review the tape. Consider important concepts such as communication, the role of culture (if you think this is applicable), and your personal values of cleanliness in developing your response.

# Patient Autonomy

A home care patient is experiencing pain secondary to surgery for head and neck cancer. She takes a liquid narcotic in suspension form. Her doctor ordered 2 teaspoons q 4h, prn pain, and gave orders to the home care nurse to titrate the dose to the patient's pain level. The home care nurse is to report on the patient's pain level and response to analgesics every week. Given the patient's condition and level of pain and previous response to analgesics, there is no fear of addiction in this patient.

The home care nurse has explained the treatment plan to the patient, and she concurs with the analgesia plan. However, the patient will not measure the amount of medication she takes each time. The nurse volunteered to "prepour" doses of medication and the patient refused this, too. Every time the home care nurse visits, the patient reports that she takes a "couple of swigs" and that it relieves the pain. She doesn't see the need to make a detailed record of her use of medication because the system she is using works. "If it ain't broke, don't fix it . . ." she repeatedly tells the home care nurse.

## CRITICAL THINKING ACTIVITY

**Using all of your nursing knowledge, creativity, and skill in dealing with patients, design a program that will be agreeable to this patient and still meet the nursing need of documenting episodes of pain and how much medication was needed for relief of pain.**

You must consider your legal and ethical role as a nurse in suggesting the alternatives to this problem. You must also consider The Patient's Bill of Rights and the ideal of patient autonomy. Your duty as a nurse directs you to provide the best care possible for this patient. In this case, you must allow the patient to manage her care and also provide supervision of her analgesic use so that proper titration can occur.

## HINTS HINTS HINTS HINTS HINTS

You may want to start with a group discussion of the issue. You can use clustering to identify the key concepts here. Refer to your fundamentals text or other material for a list of the ethical and legal principles involved in this case.

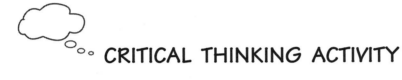

# Design the Best Patient Gown

Patient gowns never cover enough! In addition, they can interfere with patient care such as changing intravenous lines and other tubes. The patients lie on them and they can get all rolled up underneath a patient and create a mess when it is time to roll the patient from side to side. It seems that whatever job there is to do, the gown poses an obstacle to getting it done quickly and efficiently. In response to this problem, many gowns now come with snaps on the sleeves to help with IV changes. Some come with a pocket in the front to hold telemetry monitors. What else would improve a hospital gown?

## CRITICAL THINKING ACTIVITY

**Design a patient gown that is affordable, functional, and appropriate to meet the patient's needs.** Consider all the uses of the hospital gown. Remember that your gown will be used by patients in the obstetric unit, the surgical unit, the medical unit, and in critical care.

Consider what material the gown should be made of. Are there local fire or other regulations that mandate a certain type of material? What color should it be? How about the dimensions for each size? Will there be more than one size? Remember there are financial implications for each variation you design. Cost is also an important consideration.

**Draw a picture of your patient gown and describe how it is different from the existing standard gown.**

## HINTS HINTS HINTS HINTS HINTS

Wear a patient gown yourself. Try to turn over in bed, change tubes, and eat in this gown. Where does the material bunch up? Is the gown long enough? Wide enough? Look up the current statistics on the heights and weights of Americans and note how current gowns compare with their various sizes.

# A Fence or An Ambulance

## Joseph Malins

"Twas a dangerous cliff, as they freely confessed,
Though to walk near its crest was so pleasant;
Not over its terrible edge there had slipped
A duke and full many a peasant.
So the people said something would have to be done,
But their projects did not at all tally;
Some said, "Put a fence around the edge of the cliff,"
Some, "An ambulance down in the valley."

But the cry for the ambulance carried the day,
For it spread through the neighboring city;
A fence may be useful or not it is true,
But each heart became brimful of pity
For those who slipped over that dangerous cliff;
And the dwellers in highway and alley
Gave pounds or gave pence, not to put up a fence,
But an ambulance down in the valley.

"For the cliff is all right, if you're careful," they said,
"And, if folks even slip and are dropping,
It isn't the slipping that hurts them so much,
As the shock down below when they're stopping."
So day after day, as these rescuers sally
To pick up the victims who fell off the cliff,
With their ambulances down in the valley.

Then an old sage remarked:"It's a marvel to me
That people give far more attention
To repairing results than to stopping the cause,
When they'd much better aim at prevention.
Let us stop at its source all this mischief," cried he,
"Come, neighbors and friends, let us rally;
If the cliff we will fence we might almost dispense
With the ambulance down in the valley."

"Oh he's a fanatic," the others rejoined,
"Dispense with the ambulance? Never!
He'd dispense with all charities, too, if he could;
No! No! We'll support them forever.
Aren't we picking up folks just as fast as they fall?
And shall this man dictate to us? Shall he?
Why should people of sense stop to put up a fence,
While the ambulance works in the valley?"

But a sensible few, who are practical too,
Will not bear with such nonsense much longer;
They believe that prevention is better than cure,
And their party will soon be the stronger.
Encourage them then, with your purse, voice and pen,
And while other philanthropists dally,
They will scorn all pretense and put up a stout fence
On the cliff that hangs over the valley.

Better guide well the young than reclaim them when old,
For the voice of true wisdom is calling,
"To rescue the fallen is good, but 'tis best
To prevent other people from falling."
Better close up the source of temptation and crime
Than deliver from dungeon or galley;
Better put up a fence round the top of the cliff
Than an ambulance down in the valley.

 CRITICAL THINKING ACTIVITY

What is the poet trying to communicate about people? Can you relate his advice "Better guide well the young than reclaim them when old" to any health care issues? **Describe a real life health care situation for which this poem is a metaphor.** Be sure to clearly relate the "ambulance down in the valley" and the "fence around the top of the cliff." Who are the townsfolk crying for the ambulance and the fence? Who is the old sage that gets people to rethink the situation and opt for prevention?

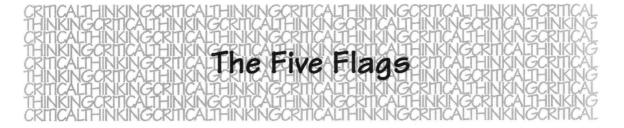

# The Five Flags

Review the description of *The Five Flags.*

We all need to develop the skill of noticing disharmony within our *OWN* mind and body. The "bodymind" will send out signals or flags when there is a problem. They can be used to diagnose a problem, or put another way, to identify a *stress reaction.* They are **positive**! They give you a chance to correct a small issue before it becomes serious. It is important for nursing students (and nurses) to constantly be aware of how patient care, school, and the demands of life impact **them.** We spend a lot of time caring for others. We need to begin early on to treat ourselves with the same care we give to our patients!

Five flags to indicate a stress reaction include:

1. Breath: When does your breathing go from full deep breaths to more rapid, labored, chest-centered breathing?

2. Movement: Changes in movements that indicate stress reactions can be obvious or subtle. They range from an obvious pulling back to a squint, a tight grasp on a pen, turning away, or other movements that indicate disharmony with what is going on.

3. Posture: This is usually a trend, rather than one movement, as in #2. You may want to look at pictures of yourself to see what postural cues you can identify. Examples include uneven shoulders, chest caved in, or one side of your jaw bulging more than the other.

4. Speech patterns: There are two components of this flag. Speech includes both the tone of the spoken word and the word itself. Was there a conversation in which you kept repeating the same thing? In which your voice changed, indicating some problems? Or were there other related cues—for example, an inability to talk at all?

5. Attitude: Includes all of the above.

From *At the Speed of Life* by Hendricks and Hendricks. Bantam Publishers. ISBN 0-553-07322-2

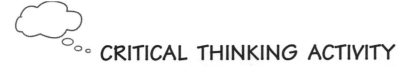

# CRITICAL THINKING ACTIVITY

**How can you add more *thinking* to the reactions you have under stressful conditions? What cues does your body give you to help your conscious mind, and what can you do to help your body and mind communicate better?**

Think back to a time this quarter or semester when you experienced a significant change in these sensations during a stressful event. Fully describe the incident, including events that led up to it, what occurred during the incident, and what you did to resolve the issue(s) that brought on the flags.

Consider ways that you may be able to use your new insight into the "flags" from your body that signal the *beginning* of a stressful reaction. Is there an early warning flag that you can use to alert your conscious mind to a pending stress reaction? How might you integrate this into daily life?

# Degrees of Separation

Words and thoughts often have small degrees of difference in their meanings and intent. Notions of what the truth is are often affected by culture, motivation, spiritual traditions, circumstance, and life events. Look at this list of words; they are in no particular order:

- Lie
- Slander
- Rumor
- Guess
- Fib
- Theory
- Half truth
- Truth

- Fiction
- Speculation
- Conjecture
- Projection
- Fact
- Opinion
- "Little white lie"

 CRITICAL THINKING ACTIVITY

**Describe the relative and absolute differences and similarities between these words.**

Draw a line across a page and line these words up with the degree of truth on the right side and the degree of falsity on the left side. Place the words accordingly along this line. Make sure that the words seem to be placed next to each other, with the smallest degrees of difference in their meaning, so that the words at each end are opposites.

Then draw another line under that one and mark the degrees to which the use of each term can prove hurtful or beneficial in any given situation. Although the terms at both end of the line are the opposites, do they have the same or different ability to hurt an individual's feeling?

Have a discussion about the significance of these terms in nursing. Is it ever okay to tell a patient a "little white lie?" Does the truth hurt? Can or should the truth be avoided sometimes?

# Legal Responsibility

With the major emphasis in downsizing and restructuring health care to be financially successful, issues of quality nursing care come up frequently. One common issue related to quality nursing care is medication errors.

To some degree, medication errors are inevitable because no one is perfect. When a medication error occurs, it is imperative that research is done into the causes and contributing factors of the error so that systems can be redesigned to prevent future errors of the same kind.

In a downsized work environment, medication errors may increase due to limited staffing with licensed nursing personnel. It is important that nurses work to be alert to medication errors caused by mistakes on the part of nursing colleagues and mistakes that result out of an understaffed environment. And that information regarding understaffing be included in final reports about medication errors.

## CRITICAL THINKING ACTIVITY

**Reflect on this question: How would I know if a medication error is a result of a nursing colleague's mistake or a result of an understaffed nursing unit?**

You are a nursing supervisor, and you want to research a medication that was omitted during a change of shift period. What questions are you going to ask? Who will you look to for information? Will it only be nursing personnel on the unit where the error occurred, or will you look beyond the obvious?

Because you are responsible for staffing according to level of care, you know that there is never *more* staff than is necessary. Often it is just enough to be adequate or slightly below what is necessary. **Does this mean there is an excuse for an error?**

# System Versus Individual

The late, William Deming, noted quality expert, said that we need to focus on systems rather than individual problems. He believed that only 15% of all the problems in organizations were related to individuals. The other 85% of organizational problems were related to the organization's systems for getting the work done.

## CRITICAL THINKING ACTIVITY

Look at the health care facility where you are working now. What problems are you most concerned about? They may not be the most important problems the facility or agency faces. It is important to identify a problem you feel strongly about. Is it one that focuses on quality patient care, confidentiality, interpersonal relations, or how health care workers communicate?

Draw a diagram explaining the problem. Be sure to identify all the individuals involved in the problem and possible solutions. Note where there are breakdown in values, policies and relationships among workers and patients in the system.

**Propose a solution to the problem using your own knowledge of the law, ethics, your own values and spiritual tradition.**

## HINTS HINTS HINTS HINTS HINTS

Be sure to pick a problem that is easily identified and described. For instance, there are problems like the patient's family being rushed to say goodbye after the patient dies, nurse's gossip about each other during breaks, or other problem. A very common complaint in hospitals is that procedures are never done on time. Patients wait and wait for their turn to go to other departments for procedures or for their pain medication. These are other examples of common systems issues.

# Qualities of Followership

Much research and discussion in organizations are related to the qualities of a good leader. Millions of dollars has gone into interviewing employees and managers to find out what constitutes the essential qualities of outstanding leadership. Even more money has gone into training and educating individuals on developing these qualities and skills. Yet one point is often missing. A good leader functions best when there are good "followers" in the organization.

There are some important qualities of the followers or subordinates to good leaders. The purpose of this activity is to identify those traits.

No matter how talented an individual leader may be, there will always be times when that person's skill is weak in some areas and he or she will need to go to others for assistance.

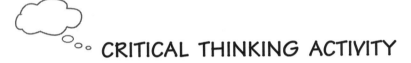

## CRITICAL THINKING ACTIVITY

**Develop a comprehensive list of qualities of good followers.** Good followers are not servants, they are not people who do as they are told.

Look at yourself and your own followership style. How do you approach new situations in which you are not in control? Can you be counted on to be a part of the team?

**Write a paper describing your own followership skills and one area that needs improvement.** Describe at least one situation in which you demonstrated superior followership skills.

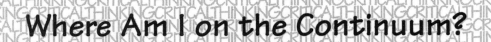

# Where Am I on the Continuum?

We are all complex creations with personalities that are collections of values. In different environments we can and do react differently, given our attention, energy, and involvement in any given situations. Consider this list of personality traits (they are lifted in no particular order):

- stubborn

- naive

- arrogant

- pathologically stubborn

- confident

- shy

- convincing

- closed minded

- timid

- self-righteous

- courageous

- bold

 **CRITICAL THINKING ACTIVITY**

Draw a line on a sheet of paper. Put the words that indicate the least amount of self-confidence on the left side of the paper and the most amount on the right side. Be careful to line the words up in continuous degrees of less or greater intensity.

**Once you have done this, describe yourself in a situation for EACH of these traits.** We cannot be naive all the time, just like we cannot be stubborn all the time. Where do you see yourself on this continuum most of the time? Ask others to share their perceptions with you.

**Prepare a paper describing the insight gained from this experience**

# Differences Between Men and Women

Women and men lead different lives. Many of the differences lead to quality of life issues. Much of this difference is based on whether an individual is a woman or man. In nursing, an essentially female profession, the impact of leading a qualitatively different life than a man is a central focus of fairness in work, governance, wages, promotion, and leadership.

The issue can be examined through a number of different "lenses." A lense in this sense is a way of focusing your attention on a particular issue. Some of the significant questions related to the topic of why are women and men treated differently are:

> Why do most professions have a dominant gender? For example, chief executive officers of major corporations are essentially white males.

> nursing has a long history of being performed by women of all classes, and status levels. However, the Knights of Pillar were both fighters and nurses.

> Why are men re-entering nursing now after a long period of being performed exclusively by women?

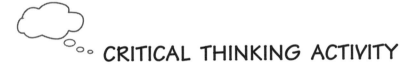 **CRITICAL THINKING ACTIVITY**

Spend a day on your unit noticing the following after observing men and women

Who is most likely to answer call lights?

Who is most likely to help another staff member clean up a patient who is incontinent?

Who answers the phone when there are several people around when it rings?

Discuss your findings with at least one other student. Present your "findings" to your class. Try to add in your own thoughts about whether the behaviors are related to gender, the situation, culture, or other factors.

# Letter of Complaint

Businesses, including educational institutions need to be aware of problem related to the service and maintenance of the products they make. In the course of providing education to future nursing students, leaders in the department need to know when there are problems. Unfortunately, discussion of problems is often associated with outbursts of uncontrolled emotions. In situations in which there are strong emotions, the actual problem can get "lost" in the high energy created in tense situations.

## CRITICAL THINKING ACTIVITY

Take some time to think about experiences you have had at the school you are attending that did not result in a positive outcome. Further reflect on ways that the situation could have been improved. What alternatives do you see now?

**After a period of reflection, write a letter of complaint, better called a letter of information or feedback, about your experience.** Address the letter to the individual responsible for the department operations or personnel involved in the situation you have selected. Build your case as a judge would build a case in a court of law. Fully explain your situation, consider alternative points of view, and give at least one suggestion for a solution.

Share your letters in class, and identify others with a similar experience. Consider rewriting letters as groups if there are similar experiences among class members.

Then deliver your letter to the appropriate individual, and work to get your suggestion implemented.

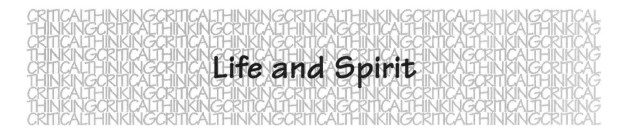

# Life and Spirit

Nursing has a long and proud herstory of integrating the care for the sick with spiritual fulfillment. For many nurses, even today, the profession of nursing cannot be separated from their personal faith. Consider these statements:

> "My daily life is my temple and religion," Kahlil Gibran
>
> "My religion is kindness," His Holiness the Fourteenth Dalai Lama
>
> "Organize your life to act out your religion," Florence Nightingale

How does your faith, spiritual tradition, or religion inform your nursing? What sacred values do you have that are demonstrated in your nursing?

Do you see any potential conflict with your own beliefs and those of the facilities you have worked in so far?

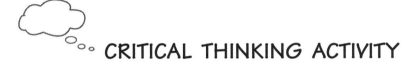

## CRITICAL THINKING ACTIVITY

**Prepare a diagram/concept map that shows two of your central spiritual beliefs and how they are demonstrated in your values as a nurse.**

Copy the diagram on to an overhead transparency, and share with your class.

Have some students takes notes and prepare a diagram that describes the common themes among class members.

# CRITICAL THINKING ACTIVITIES RELATED TO AGING

# Come to Me

## Sue Elkind

Description: Come to me looking

As you did fifty years ago

Arms outstretched

And I waiting

Virgin again

In white that changes

To splashes of roses

As we lie together.

Come to me smiling again

With your mortar and pestle

And vitamin pills

Because I am given to colds

And coughs that wrack us both.

Oh! Come to me again

And I will be there

Waiting with withered hands

Gnarled fingers

That leave their marks

Of passion on your back

## CRITICAL THINKING ACTIVITY

Read this poem several times. After reading it and reflecting on the deep emotions expressed in the poem, complete a one-page list of interview questions that you could ask the author to elicit more information about her sexual feelings. **Write a short paragraph describing what you feel a normal sexual relationship would be for a healthy, 75-year-old woman.**

# Ecclesiastes 3:1–11

Description: To everything there is a season, and a time to every purpose under the heaven:

> A time to be born, and a time to die;
> A time to plant, and a time to pluck up that which is planted;
>
> A time to kill, and a time to heal;
> A time to break down, and a time to build up;
>
> A time to weep, and a time to laugh;
> A time to mourn, and a time to dance;
>
> A time to cast away stones, and a time to gather stones together;
> A time to embrace, and a time to refrain from embracing;
>
> A time to seek, and a time to lose;
> A time to keep, and a time to cast away;
>
> A time to rend, and a time to sew;
> A time to keep silence, and a time to speak;
>
> A time to love and a time to hate;
> A time for war, and a time for peace.

## CRITICAL THINKING ACTIVITY

**Consider these basic principles in life.** Sit quietly and feel the power of their simple truths. Compare and contrast one of these lines.

**Think back on your experience during the last few days of providing nursing care.** Did you experience a day in which you had a "time to mourn, and a time to dance?" Were you able to mourn or dance in your day? Were you able to recognize the differences in experience during the same day? **Rewrite the "script" of that day to include both sides of emotion.** Share your reflections in a group. What themes emerge? What can be done about it?

# H I N T S H I N T S H I N T S H I N T S H I N T S

Health care providers sometimes become "numb" to the suffering of others around them. Not because they don't care, but because there can be a tremendous personal cost to acknowledging the many losses our patients endure. As a result of becoming numb to pain, one becomes numb to the dance.

# The Passionate Pilgrim

Crabbed age and youth cannot live together:
Youth is full of pleasure, age is full of care;
Youth is like a summer morn, age like winter weather;
Youth like summer brave, age like winter weather;
Youth is full of sport, age's breath is short;
Youth is nimble, age is lame;
Age I do abhor thee; youth I do adore thee;
O, my love, my love is young!
Age, I do defy thee: O, sweet shepherd, hie thee
For methinks thou stay'st too long.

## CRITICAL THINKING ACTIVITY

**Explore what it is like for The Passionate Pilgrim** to grow old. Describe your impression of the aged person's self-image in this passage. List five interview questions (in proper question format) that you would ask the aged person in the passage to obtain further information about his feelings regarding aging.

**Derive five nursing diagnoses from the aged person's thoughts.** Make sure they are in the correct format, using the three-part statement (problem, etiology, and defining characteristics).

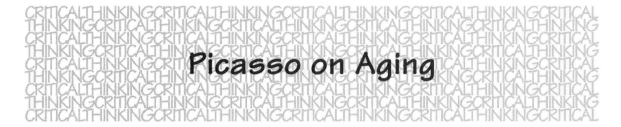

# Picasso on Aging

Pablo Picasso said,"It takes a very long time to become young."

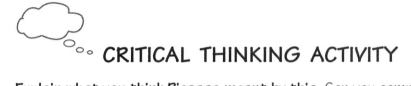

## CRITICAL THINKING ACTIVITY

**Explain what you think Picasso meant by this.** Can you compare the idea(s) behind this quote with any of the standard developmental theories you have studied? Does Erikson's stage of "Ego Integrity vs. Despair" fit with this quote? What other developmental theories are pertinent?

If you were having a conversation with Picasso, how would you respond? **Write down the next line, in response to Picasso's statement.**

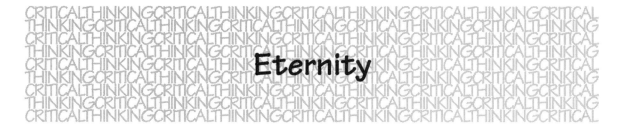

# Eternity

## William Blake

He who bends to himself a joy
Does the winged life destroy;
But he who kisses the joy as it flies
Lives in eternity's sunrise

This is an often-repeated verse in nursing homes and social groups focused on aging. It seems to give many people, especially older people, a great deal of inspiration in their lives.

 **CRITICAL THINKING ACTIVITY**

Share this passage with three older people you know. Analyze their answers for similarities and differences. Did any of them seem to have underlying assumptions that make this verse seem hopeful to them? What does this verse tell you about being joyful in life?

**Prepare a written paper comparing your answers with those of your older informants.**

# A Tribute to the Elderly

## Denise Stone

We see them as children
Crazy
And so very, very old.

But had we known them years ago
The stories they could have told.
Think of all the knowledge that they carry
That we could have possessed.
But as we see them now,
With their weak and fragile minds
You never would have guessed.

But as they are
We sometimes forget
That they are people too.
With feelings and compassion
Just like you and me.

So remember when you are with them
That this is not a game.
For as time goes on
We all grow old
And we shall be the same.

This poem was written by Miss Stone, who is a personal care attendant and a nursing assistant student. She writes from a deep sense of commitment to the frail elderly.

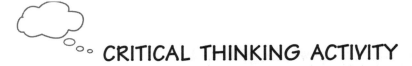

# CRITICAL THINKING ACTIVITY

Western society has some deep-seated aversions to growing old. Nurses often regard long-term care facilities as depressing places. What is your idea? How do Miss Stone's ideas compare with yours?

Do you aspire to work exclusively with the elderly? What would the experience of working in a long-term care facility be like for you? What would be the advantages and disadvantages? Do you see it as an interesting and fun place? Could you see spending your nursing career there?

**Prepare a paper on your views, relating your ideas to the words in Miss Stone's poem.** Every time you identify a feeling about the aged, look deeply at that feeling for the underlying assumptions and discuss those. If you think working in long-term care is depressing, reflect on that thought. What specifically about long-term care is depressing as it relates to your life?

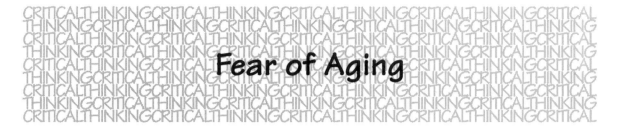

# Fear of Aging

In many societies, there is a fear of aging that is often unexamined prior to becoming older. The purpose of this activity is to identify some of your own concerns about aging and also to identify some of the joys associated with aging.

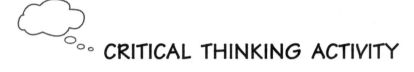

## CRITICAL THINKING ACTIVITY

Look around at older people in your family and in your community. What do you think when you look at them? How old do you expect to be at the time of your death? In what physical and mental condition do you expect to be at the time of your death?

**Make two lists. First list the concerns you have about aging. In the second list, describe those things that getting older gives you "permission" to do.**

Share your results with a small group and compile your group's list of advantages of growing older.

# HINTS HINTS HINTS HINTS HINTS

The idea is to see aging in its entirety. There are disadvantages but also many, many advantages to aging. The list of advantages should be at least as long, and probably longer than the list of disadvantages.

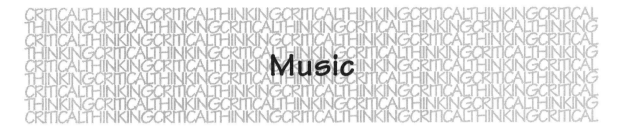

# Music

## Amy Lowell

The neighbour sits in his window and plays the flute.
From my bed I can hear him.
And the round notes flutter and tap about the room,
And hit against each other,
Blurring to unexpected chords.
It is very beautiful,
With the little flute-notes all about me,
In the darkness.

In the daytime,
The neighbour eats bread and onions with one hand
And copies music with the other.
He is fat and has a bald head,
So I do not look at him,
But run quickly past his window.
There is always the sky to look at,
Or the water in the well!

But when night comes and he plays his flute,
I think of him as a young man,
With gold seals hanging from his watch,
And blue coat with silver buttons.
As I lie on my bed
The flute-notes push against my ears and lips,
And I go to sleep dreaming.

 ## CRITICAL THINKING ACTIVITY

Write two versus of a poem in which the man, who is the subject of this poem, writes about the *woman* who is his neighbor.

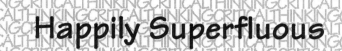

# Happily Superfluous

Noted Jungian analyst Helen Luke wrote eloquently about aging.

One of her books talked about the goals of old age. One goal was to "become happily superfluous."

 **CRITICAL THINKING ACTIVITY**

**Explore what this means to you.** Is it "right" to see some members of society as superfluous, whether or not they want to be regarded this way?

# You Are Old, Father William

## Lewis Carroll

"You are old, Father William," the young man said,
"And your hair has become very white;
And yet you incessantly stand on your head—
Do you think, at your age, it is right?"

"In my youth," Father William replied to his son,
"I feared it might injure the brain;
But now that I'm perfectly sure I have none,
Why, I do it again and again."

"You are old, said the youth," and your jaws are too weak
For anything other than suet;
Yet you finished the goose, with the bones and the beak—
Pray, how did you manage to do it?"

"In my youth," said his father, "I took to the law,
And argued each case with my wife;
And the muscular strength, which it gave to my jaw,
Has lasted the rest of my life."

 CRITICAL THINKING ACTIVITY

**Prepare a paper describing the underlying assumptions of both the father and the son.** Compare and contrast the lines from this classic verse. Conclude your paper with a suggestion of how you think the son will age with this father as a role model.

# Chinese Old Man

There was a Chinese man living with his son on the family farm. The man was too old and weak to do more than sit on the porch and watch the young family members work.

One day the son wheeled a pine box up to the porch and told his father to get in. He went on to say that the father wasn't any good anymore since he could not work and contribute to the family. The father complied immediately and closed the lid on himself. As the son wheeled his father and the box toward the cliff where he was going to throw them over the edge, the son heard a knock on the box.

The son stopped and opened the box and asked his father what he wanted. The father replied, "I can understand what you are doing and why you are doing it. I just have one suggestion. Why don't you just throw me over the edge and save the box? Your son will need it someday."

 CRITICAL THINKING ACTIVITY

What was your first thought after realizing the point of this story? What do you think the son did after the father's last comment?

**Complete a paper describing your reaction to this story.** In the paper, describe the underlying assumptions about aging that were demonstrated. In addition, compare this story with Western traditions and identify cultural differences and similarities.

# CHAPTER

# 3

# CRITICAL THINKING ACTIVITIES RELATED TO DEATH AND DYING

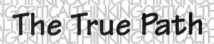

# The True Path

Description:

Just before Ninakawa passed away, the Zen master Ikkyu visited him. "Shall I lead you on?" Ikkyu asked.

Ninakawa replied: "I came here alone and I go alone. What help could you be to me?"

Ikkyu answered: "If you think you really come and go, that is your delusion. Let me show you the path on which there is no coming or going."

With his words, Ikkyu had revealed the path so clearly that Ninakawa smiled and passed away.

This is from a book on Buddhist (Zen) stories, *Zen Flesh, Zen Bones,* compiled by Paul Reps. This Buddhist passage describes the "coming and going" associated with reincarnation. There is also another important Buddhist idea in this passage—that of nirvana, or buddha-hood. It is described in"Let me show you the path on which there is no coming or going."

 CRITICAL THINKING ACTIVITY

**Explain how this passage compares with your ideas about death.** Do you see it as a coming and going? How does your spiritual belief system compare with this one? What did you feel when you read the last line ". . . he smiled and passed away?" Is that what happens in the United States at the time of death? Why or why not?

**Draw a diagram or map to illustrate the comparison between your beliefs regarding life and death and those presented in this passage.** Share your ideas in a small group.

# The Man Who Was Aware of Death

## Bayazid of Bistam

There was once a dervish who embarked upon a sea journey. As the other passengers on the ship came aboard one by one, they saw him and —as was the custom—asked him for a piece of advise. All the dervish would do was say the same thing to each of them; he seemed merely to be repeating one of those formulas that each dervish makes the object of his attention from time to time.

The formula was: 'Try to be aware of death, until you know what death is.' Few of the travelers felt particularly attracted to this admonition.

Presently a terrible storm blew up. The crew and the passengers alike fell upon their knees imploring God to save the ship. They alternately screamed in terror, gave themselves up for lost, and hoped wildly for succor. All of this time, the dervish sat quietly, reflective, reacting not at all to the movement and the scenes that surrounded him.

Eventually the buffeting stopped, the sea and sky were calm, and the passengers became aware of how serene the dervish had been throughout the episode.

One of them asked him: "Did you not realize that during the frightful tempest there was nothing more solid than a plank between us all and death?"

"Oh yes indeed," answered the dervish. "I knew that at sea it is always thus. I also realized, however, that I had often reflected when I was on land that, in the normal course of events, there is even less between us and death".

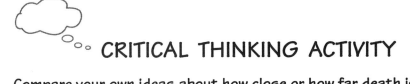 CRITICAL THINKING ACTIVITY

**Compare your own ideas about how close or how far death is with those of the dervish.** How do you feel about his idea that after the storm, ". . . there is even less between us and death"?

**Rewrite this short story and substitute your own ideas about death in place of the dervish's.**

# H I N T S H I N T S H I N T S H I N T S H I N T S

You may now be as aware of death as the dervish. The idea is to summarize and apply your own ideas of how far or near death is so you can reflect on your ideas of death. No matter what area of health care you work in, death will be a part of it. Your own reflections on death will help or hinder your work with patients and their families.

# My Father At Eighty-Five

## Robert Bly

His large ears
Hear everything.
A hermit wakes
And sleeps in a hut
Underneath
His gaunt cheeks.
His eyes blue, alert,
Disappointed,
And suspicious,
Complain I
Do not bring him
The same sorts of
Jokes the nurses
Do. He is a bird
Waiting to be fed,—
Mostly beak—an eagle
Or a vulture, or
The Pharaoh's servant
Just before death.
My arm on the bedrail
Rests there, relaxed,
With new love. All
I know of the Troubadours
I bring to this bed.
I do not want
Or need to be shamed
by him any longer.
The general of shame
Has discharged
Him, and left him
In this small provincial
Egyptian town.
If I do not wish
To shame him, then
Why not love him?

His long hands,
Large, veined,
Capable, can still
Retain hold of what
He wanted. But
Is that what he
Desired? Some
Powerful engine
Of desire goes on
Turning inside his body,
He never phrased
What he desired,
And I am
His son.

## CRITICAL THINKING ACTIVITY

This is a poem Robert Bly composed at his father's side in a hospital bed during his last days. Read it several times. You want to try and discover the nature of the relationship between the father and son. **Your goal is to incorporate the son's feelings regarding his father into the nursing plan of care.**

What are the issues the son has identified? Do you think the father and son have had a healthy relationship during the past years? Look at Mr. Bly's (the poet's) use of terms and try to see his descriptions of the effects of illness, the hospital environment, and the relationship between his father and the nurses caring for him. Analyze at least four lines of the poem. Compare your experience as a nurse with the experience of this son. How can you help him say goodbye to his dying father? Does it seem that there is anything left undone?

# The Patient Who Didn't Die

Description of problem: A hospice patient shoots himself in the head, but does not die. Instead he is found by his family shortly after trying to kill himself and is transferred to the local community hospital. He is now in intensive care, on a ventilator. You are the nurse assigned to care for him this shift.

His physician approaches you, obviously distressed over this turn of events. He can barely talk, he is so overcome with grief over the patient's attempt to kill himself. The physician talks of feeling frustrated and inadequate as a healer. He wonders what he could have done to help the patient's suffering during the last weeks of his life.

The patient's wife is in the waiting room and wants to know what is going on with her husband. It is time to help the wife answer the question: What now? The physician is not in any emotional condition to speak with the wife. So it is up to you.

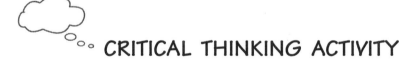 CRITICAL THINKING ACTIVITY

**Explore how to help the wife decide what to do next. Write a script of the conversation between you and the patient's wife.** Include the beginning of the conversation and continue to a resolution of where the patient should go to die and what level of care he should receive. What do you say? Where do you start the conversation? What will the wife's response be?

Be sure to explain the emotions, facial looks, body language, and tone of speech. You may want to do this in the form of a poem, story, or actual script.

# H I N T S HINTS H I N T S HINTS H I N T S

Consider The Patient's Bill of Rights, The Hospice Patient's Bill of Rights, your state's laws regarding terminal patient care, your State's Board of Registered Nursing Practice Act, and any other appropriate regulations in making your script.

# Buddhist Perspective on Death

## Soygal Rinpoche

There would be no chance at all of getting to know death if it happened only once. But fortunately, life is nothing but a continuing dance of birth and death, a dance of change. Every time I hear the rush of a mountain stream, or the waves crashing on the shore, or my own heartbeat, I hear the sound of impermanence. These changes, these small deaths, are our living links with death. They are death's pulses, death's heartbeat, prompting us to let go of all things we cling to.

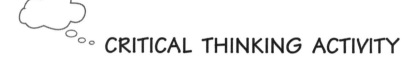 CRITICAL THINKING ACTIVITY

Sit in a quiet place and reflect on this passage from Soygal Rinpoche's *Glimpse After Glimpse*; this is the passage for June 12. **Consider the following questions: Where do people go after they die? What can one do on earth to affect where he or she goes after death?**

Use a mapping or cluster method to describe your belief system. This is NOT an exercise in describing your religious beliefs. It is an exercise in facing death, and thinking about how you will answer the dying patients who will be asking YOU this question (many, many times during your nursing career).

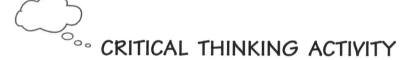

# Funeral Planning Brochure

Many families of patients who died during the course of a hospitalization report that they wished they had made the funeral arrangements before their loved one died. Over and over again family members report that this was the most difficult thing they had to do. Waiting until after the death made them more vulnerable to the funeral director (although the majority are very honest people). There was just so much else to do after the death that the funeral planning made the first days unbearable. Lastly, they did not have an opportunity to ask their loved one what he or she wanted for the funeral.

Nurses can help family members of dying patients by encouraging them to go to the funeral home and make arrangements before their loved one dies. This will also give the family members a chance to bring up the subject of death and start the grieving process with their loved one.

## CRITICAL THINKING ACTIVITY

**Identify how the nurse should bring up the subject of funeral planning with the patient's family before the patient dies.**

Design a patient education handout on funeral planning. Make sure your handout includes information on why it should be done before the patient dies, where to go for funeral planning, and tips on bringing up the subject with the patient.

Next write a policy for the department in which the brochure will be used. Then design an inservice for the staff. Be sure to include a role play of a staff member and a family member discussing the need to go to a funeral home before the patient dies.

# I Do, I Don't

You have been working in home health care with a client who has had pancreatic cancer for several months. Although the client is in her fifties and in relatively good health otherwise, the cancer is taking its toll. She is now bedbound. She sleeps most of the day. When you visit she usually wakes up and is able to share some stories about her life. You learn that she has lived with a man whom she calls her "husband" for 30 years. But they are not married. They have grown children and by all outward appearances they are a successfully married couple. Your client's dying wish is that they be married. She tells you over and over that this is the one "undone" job she has.

This seems like an easy job to you. The client is clearly dying and any official marriage would be a short one. You call her partner at work and meet him for coffee one afternoon, not in the client's home. You are a little nervous and excited about this chance to really grant your client her dying wish. You spell out your plan to the "husband." You have already contacted a local minister who is willing to do the ceremony for free in the client's home. All your client's partner has to say is "I do."

His answer is swift: "No."

All the same reservations the client had told you he gave her are laid out in front of you. The bottom line is that there will be no marriage. You are heartbroken and grateful you have not shared your plan with the client.

After going back to the office you share your disappointment with a colleague. She has a new suggestion: why not get a "fake" minister and have the couple married? The "minister" won't be legally authorized to do the ceremony, so the client's partner will not be legally married. His fears will be eliminated, and she will die thinking she was married.

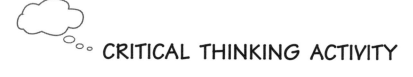 **CRITICAL THINKING ACTIVITY**

Now the marriage is back in your lap. Do you suggest this plan to the husband? Do you just forget the whole thing? As the nurse, is it important to address this woman's dying wish? What feelings do you have toward the man who would not marry a woman after

30 years and several children? How do your feelings affect your decision to proceed or not proceed? Would it make any difference to you if this patient was not dying?

**Either write a letter to the client's partner requesting his cooperation in this marriage or perform a role play in which you talk with the client's partner to show your resolution of the situation.**

# What to Say Next. . . .

Two weeks ago, Mrs. Alison was told she has cancer. Then several biopsies demonstrated that she had extensive unresectable cancer. Chemotherapy would not likely be of any help, because the cancer has invaded several organs and her bones. Mrs. Alison reports, "I only felt like had the flu and my arthritis was acting up . . ." The news was devastating to her.

Her family consists of one son who lives in the same town and one son in prison on a sentence that will last several decades. Upon hearing the news, the son who lives close to her moves in with her. He has never provided any personal care to anyone, let alone his mother. She has always been the strong one in the family.

Her need for care becomes more intense in the week since hearing the news. Although she can still get out of bed, it is getting harder and harder. Her son seems to be trying to keep all of his objections and concerns to himself. That is until one morning. . . .

The patient awoke late that morning. She had been up late the night before, trying to get her pain under control. She could still give herself medication and eat on her own, if her son prepared the food, which he had been doing. This morning, he did not answer her when she called for him. She could hear the television in the living room and she guessed he might have fallen asleep, since he had stayed up with her most of the night. Several hours passed and she continued to call for him periodically, but he never answered.

Finally, her pain was getting so intense she needed to get another bottle, which was kept in the kitchen. She decided to walk to the kitchen to get the medication. After slipping out of bed, she fell to the floor, and simply crawled as best she could. As she passed the living room on the way to the kitchen, she found her son, collapsed on the floor. He did not answer her when she called to him. When she shook him, she feared he was dead. She called 911. . . .

When the paramedics got to the house they found that her son was dead, from an apparent overdose (of her morphine pain pills). He left a short note saying he ". . . just couldn't provide the care anymore . . .". Given her rapidly declining health, her lack of a caregiver, and the fact that her pain was out of control, she was transferred to the inpatient hospice unit.

Since her arrival at the unit she has been angry, acting out, and generally not cooperating with the nursing staff. She complains about everything done for her and calls the supervisor into her room several times to complain about "the nurses."

It's the change of shift and you are on the night shift. The patient is still awake when you do your rounds. Her admission assessment identifies her as a "night owl," so you expect her to be awake most of the shift. The rest of the patients are quiet. You have some time to go in and talk to her. But where will you start?

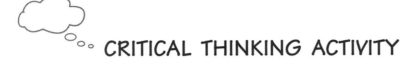 ## CRITICAL THINKING ACTIVITY

**Develop a strategy to try to build a bridge of understanding with this woman.** What are the relevant points of the description you've read? What issues do you see beyond the obvious ones? What were/are the patient's underlying assumptions about her situation?—you may find a deeper answer to her suffering by examining those. What are your assumptions about this situation? What is the role of the hospice program as a whole, and what is your role as a nurse in particular?

Consider showing your strategy in a role play with another student or students.

## HINTS HINTS HINTS HINTS HINTS

Remember, it's the night shift. It's up to you and the patient to communicate—there's no one else around!

# A Year to Live

His Holiness The Dalai Lama is often asked about his future plans. He always has the same answer: "I'm preparing for death." He is in good health and in his sixties, and shows no signs of imminent death.

Stephen Levine, a noted death expert, and his wife wrote a book about their experience of taking 1 year and living it as if it were their last one. In their book, *A Year to Live,* they explained some profound insights into the experience of living as if they had a year left:

> Living life with forgiveness and gratitude
>
> Not having time to be hurt
>
> Facing life responsibly
>
> That most people feel they are facing fears about death because they are able to submerge the fears and not think about them

Most people in the West would regard the Levine's experiment and His Holiness's preoccupation with death as unusual, perhaps inappropriate. What do you think?

## CRITICAL THINKING ACTIVITY

Here is your chance to consider what is really important in your life and to reach some profound insights about yourself. Often the process of learning that you have a year left begins with a life review. **Review what your life has been like until now.** Consider discussing this exercise with someone close to you. This can be a profound experience and is worth sharing with those you love.

**Once you have reviewed your life and are able to begin to look forward to your next year, write down the following:**

1. A list of things to do.

2. A list of things NOT to do.

Consider sharing this in small groups. Identify the similarities and differences among your group members.

# What To Do Next?

Mr. Allen was recently admitted to the medical/surgical unit. He is 56 years old and looks to be in excellent health. His skin is tanned, and he "seems too healthy" to be terminal. He is suffering from cancer of the kidney, with metastasis to his bones. He has had several surgeries over the last several years, including a nephrectomy and a bladder reconstruction. However, the cancer is spreading.

Last night Mr. Allen felt a sudden sharp pain in his left upper arm and got up to see what it was. He found that he had sustained a spontaneous pathologic fracture of his right humerus. His physician had told him that this was a possibility, so he was not totally surprised. As he started to get out of bed to get some pain medication, he fell to the floor. His left femur also fractured. Metastasis had weakened his bones, causing both fractures.

His wife awoke when she heard him hit the floor. She called 911 and he was taken to the emergency department in excruciating pain. He was given morphine sulfate until he fell asleep. However, any movement at all caused excruciating pain and caused him to awake screaming.

When you received a report on his condition, you were told by the emergency department nurse that Mr. Allen's level of orientation was deteriorating, even before the morphine was administered. The nurse told you that every time she looked into his eyes she saw "all the suffering of the world" looking back at her. No one held back the pain medication. They gave him morphine before and after they moved him. He was getting it in a continuous drip. The reality was that the extent of his disease, coupled with two pathologic fractures, was beyond what morphine could relieve.

Mr. Allen's family did not accompany him to the medical/surgical unit. They were exhausted. The emergency room nurse told you that his mother and two adult daughters accompanied him to the emergency room but left when the doctors said that they had done all they could do. The doctors offered surgery to stabilize the bones but also gave a grave warning of his probable inability to survive the surgery. If he did survive, then what? Another fracture? Then what? Mr. Allen probably has another 4 to 6 months to live, without the fractures. What can be done for him in the meantime? What are the nurses going to do for him? What is it going to be like to take care of him and his family? The staff has some time to think about it. The family has gone home to think things over. Mr. Allen was transferred to his bed, amidst his screams of pain, but he is resting now and is not scheduled for anything for a couple of hours.

The head nurse decides that the first place to start in planning his care is for each nurse to decide what she would do in this situation. There are no books to describe what the care should be. The nurses need experience, spiritual philosophy, knowledge, ethics, and values to guide them.

# CRITICAL THINKING ACTIVITY

**What would you do if you were the nurse to care for Mr. Allen and his family?** What are the nursing diagnoses that apply?—name the two most important. Is there a nursing diagnosis that fits this situation? If you had to choose surgery or no surgery, what would you decide? Why? Would your answer change if this were your father or husband? Why?

# HINTS HINTS HINTS HINTS HINTS

Remember, critical thinking is not just a matter of opinion. It is a product of reasoned judgment. What facts are available to help you with your decision?

# What Do You Say Next?

The families of our patients often find themselves wondering about the conditions of their loved ones. They may not be available when the physicians visit the patient or, for numerous reasons, they may not fully grasp the meaning of the physician's explanations. These families often turn to the nurse to fill in the gaps of information.

However, this can leave the nurse in a difficult position. This is especially true if the patient's situation is life-threatening. Consider the following scenario.

You are a senior student nurse, just ready to graduate, and you are caring for an elderly man dying of lung cancer. You first cared for him last week, and even then you realized he was not going to live much longer. You were surprised to be assigned to him again today. You've heard the nurses and doctors say that he is "living on borrowed time." Your own physical assessment confirms that he has a decreased level of consciousness, early stages of distal extremity mottling, and hypotension. He still has some urine output, and an even smaller intake of fluids by mouth.

The family recognizes you from last week as you walk in the room. They comment that they are happy to have you back because you provided such "loving care" to their loved one. You are both reassured and a little anxious about caring for him today. You wonder if this is the day he will die. After you complete your morning care, the patient's adult daughter comes up to you and with tears in her eyes asks "Is my father going to die?"

You look around. None of the registered nurses or patient's physicians are around. It is an extremely busy day on the unit, and everyone seems to be involved with their patients. What do you do? What do you say?

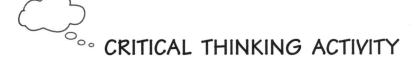

## CRITICAL THINKING ACTIVITY

**Consider how you would answer this question from a family member: "Is my father going to die?"** Think about the ramifications of both answering and not answering. How would you feel if you were the person asking the question? Where in the list of demands of nursing care does the family come in? How does the student nurse differ from the staff nurse in this situation—if at all? Does the fact that your own assessment—as a senior ready to graduate—confirms that the patient is actively dying make a difference?

Your answer should be a result of some standard of thinking. It is more than just a re-flection of your comfort level with answering this question. **What are your legal and ethical responsibilities in answering this question?**

Consider presenting your findings in a role play or script format.

# HINTS HINTS HINTS HINTS HINTS

Consult your state's Nurse Practice Act, and your texts on communication and care of the dying. You may also want to consult the hospital or the policy and procedure manual of your facility.

# Milarepa's Death Verse

Milarepa was one of the most dedicated students of the Buddha. He has a famous verse about facing death, often quoted by people who work in care of the dying. It is:

In horror of death, I took to the mountains

Again and again I meditated on the uncertainty of the hour of death,

Capturing the fortress of the deathless unending nature of mind.

Now all fear of death is over and done.

This verse reflects two certainties about death. First, we will all die. Second, no one knows when he or she will die.

It is well known that although patients and families may not speak to their health care givers about death, they are speaking to each other. The health care system in the West does not discuss death in the "light of day." Often conversations about death do not include the individual with a life-threatening condition, are whispered, and are kept short.

Although patients often fear being kept alive by machines, they do not find individuals or circumstances to discuss the alternatives in a way that does not create or enhance a sense of dread.

Reflecting on death, before death is "staring you in the face," may be one way to bring death into the conversation about life.

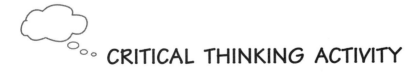 **CRITICAL THINKING ACTIVITY**

**Spend 30 minutes reflecting on this verse.** Does thinking about your own death cause you a lot of discomfort? Does thinking about death decrease anxiety? Is this something you could talk to patients or clients about? Why or why not?

# As Befits a Man

## Langston Hughes

Description: I don't mind dying—
But I'd hate to die all alone!
I want a dozen pretty women
To holler, cry, and moan.

I don't mind dying
But I want my funeral to be fine:
A row of long tall mamas
Fainting, fanning, and crying.

I want a fish-tail hearse
And sixteen fish-tail cars,
A big brass band
And a whole truck load of flowers.

When they lay me down,
Down into the clay,
I want the women to holler:
Please don't take him away!
Ow-ooo-oo-o!
Don't take daddy away!

 CRITICAL THINKING ACTIVITY

Compare this view of what a funeral should be with your own view of a funeral. What are the similarities and differences? How would you approach this patient versus the person in Shakespeare's Passionate Pilgrim (see Chapter 2)?

**Prepare a brief care plan contrasting the developmental differences between the subjects of these two poetry pieces.**

CHAPTER

# 4

# CRITICAL THINKING ACTIVITIES RELATED TO NURSING ETHICS

# Ten Commandments of Nursing

Christians and Jews throughout the world lead their lives by the Ten Commandments as described in the Bible. These commandments range from 'don't lie' to 'honor your father and mother.' Buddhists throughout the world subscribe to the Four Noble Truths, such as the cause of suffering is attachment, and the Eightfold Path, which includes such behavioral guidelines as the "right speech." Social and political organizations also have codes of conduct and laws that govern daily life. These codes are often a synthesis of the greater teachings or mission of the organization. They serve to educate the members about the most essential rules of the group. Consider what the "Ten Commandments of Nursing" would look like.

 CRITICAL THINKING ACTIVITY

Reflect on the essential elements of nursing and the rules of conduct that govern our profession. Each state has a practice act. Speciality organizations also have guidelines of member conduct. The facilities that nurses work at have their own sets of rules, and so on. Using clustering or listing or group discussion, brainstorm on which essential actions and restrictions comprise nursing practice. Think about the "generic" or basic common elements of nursing—those rules that would apply no matter where a nurse worked.

**Describe your own "10 Commandments of Nursing" (or some other number).**

# HINTS HINTS HINTS HINTS HINTS

Be careful to describe enough rules to be comprehensive, but not so many that they are difficult to use. Be prepared to share these rules in class.

# How to Tell The Truth

You are a nurse in a cardiologist's office. Mr. Anderson has been coming to the office at regular, frequent intervals since he had a large anterior myocardial infarction 2 months ago. Although Mr. Anderson is only 65 years old, the heart attack left him with residual congestive heart failure and arrhythmia. You've gotten to know both Mr. and Mrs. Anderson during their visits and have assisted with his exercise stress test and other diagnostic procedures. You and the cardiologist have discussed his poor prognosis on several occasions. Mr. and Mrs. Anderson have been informed of the physician's prognosis and seem to accept an early death as a reality.

The problem is that their adult daughter, Ann, is an only child. She is getting married and wants her father to give her away. Mr. Anderson has expressly stated that he does not want anyone communicating the full extent of his condition to his daughter, who calls after every doctor's appointment to check on her father. You know that Ann loves her father very much and wants only the best for him. In talking with her, you are also aware that she does not know the extent of the myocardial damage caused by the heart attack. On this day Ann, calls and asks a specific question: "I want to set my wedding date for this time next year, to give my father plenty of time to recover from his heart attack. Do you think that is enough time for him to recover?" Ann goes on to tell you how much it means to her to have her father there. You also know that the chances that Mr. Anderson will still be alive in one year are very slim.

## CRITICAL THINKING ACTIVITY

**Given your legal, ethical, and occupational restrictions, how can you answer the question of when to have the wedding and not violate any professional guidelines?** You know that Mr. Anderson's reluctance to tell his daughter the truth is the reason for her decision to postpone the wedding past his expected length of life. Mrs. Anderson has been no help. You have expressed your concern about Ann being left out of the "information loop" to her privately, and she has indicated she will abide by Mr. Anderson's wishes of keeping Ann uninformed. First, be sure to identify the most significant legal, ethical, and occupational issues here before completing the activity.

# H I N T S H I N T S H I N T S H I N T S H I N T S

Sit and reflect on this story . . . put yourself in the place of each family member. How does it feel to be withholding the information? How does it feel to be the one calling and not getting any information? How does it feel to be the nurse who wants to nurse the entire family and help everyone say their goodbyes but can't?

# Taking Care of the Victim AND the Criminal

You are a night nurse working in a medium-sized community hospital. During your shift a young woman is brought into the intensive care unit (ICU) with multiple stab wounds, including amputation of both arms by her assailant. In addition, the assailant poured lime in her eyes and blinded her, before he left her for dead at the side of the road. A passer-by found her and called the police and paramedics. She is barely alive but is expected to survive the ordeal.

Shortly after finding the young victim, police investigating the crime were tipped off to the assailant through a routine traffic stop of the criminal, when it was found that the car he was driving was the victim's. The perpetrator tried to run away from the arresting police officers and was critically wounded.

Just after midnight the victim arrives, barely conscious but breathing on her own. You are struck by the immensity and savagery of the mutilation she has endured. The police officer assigned to monitor her condition tells you she is a runaway. They are trying to contact her mother but are having difficulty locating her.

Around 2:00 o'clock in the morning, the criminal arrives in the ICU after extensive surgery to repair the internal damage from the police gunshot wounds. He is on the ventilator, and doctors are uncertain as to whether he will live. He is too sick to be transferred to the county jail ward, so you and your staff must care for both the criminal and the victim in the same ICU.

## CRITICAL THINKING ACTIVITY

**What are your feelings about caring for the victim of a brutal and senseless crime, as well as the criminal who committed the violent acts?** Do you feel you can care for both with equal parts of caring and concern? **What does your heart tell you? What does your professional standard of conduct tell you? How do your feelings relate to professional standards?**

How are they the same? How are they different? Draw a cluster diagram illustrating the feelings you are having. Show the interrelationships between what your heart and mind are telling you, and what your professional standards tell you. Use personal symbols to further illustrate your feelings.

# HINTSHINTSHINTSHINTSHINTS

Put yourself in the criminal's place. What does it feel like to be so overcome with inner rage that mutilating a young woman seems to be at least a partial solution to your problems? What factors contributed to the development of such a violent personality?

Put yourself in the place of the victim. What does it feel like to be armless and blind after being raped and left for dead? Is there anything of comfort that has happened or is happening to you?

# Prayer of Saint Francis of Assisi

Lord, Make me an instrument of your peace.
Where there is hatred, let me sow love.
Where there is injury, pardon.
Where there is doubt, faith.
Where there is despair, hope.
Where there is darkness, light.
Where there is sadness, joy.
O Divine Master, grant that I may not so much seek
To be consoled, as to console,
To be understood, as to understand,
To be loved as to love,
For it is giving that we receive,
It is in pardoning that we are pardoned,
It is in dying that we are born to eternal life.

 ## CRITICAL THINKING ACTIVITY

Read this prayer several times. Reflect on the deeper meanings. Consider how this prayer reflects (or doesn't reflect) your values as a nurse. **Using a narrative format or a diagram, compare and contrast your role as a nurse with the ideals of this prayer.** Do you see yourself as joyful? As a consoler? As an instrument of peace?

# Answer a Simple Question!

A young Latino couple was involved in a serious auto accident. Teresa, the young woman was badly injured, and her husband was killed. She is an only child. Her parents flew across the country to stay by her side as soon as they heard about the accident. One of them is always at her side.

Teresa's parents are concerned and cooperative in her care. They are anxious to help her in any way possible. Except for one thing. They forbid the staff to tell their daughter that her husband has been killed. Her father has made it clear that he intends to tell her, but he will know the right time and prays about this everyday. Their rationale is that he is already dead, and Teresa's health would be placed in great jeopardy if she were to be told. Teresa's mother is a nurse, and her father is an engineer. They are articulate about the ethical issues of disclosure and consent. Their daughter is over 18 years of age.

You have just started your usual evening shift. It is around 5:00 PM. Teresa is more alert than usual; her vital signs are stable. Teresa stops you during your physical exam and asks "Where is my husband?" Both of her parents are at the bedside, and they jump to "attention" at Teresa's question. She has not asked this question before. You are caught by surprise, too. This is the moment you and the rest of the staff have dreaded since Teresa was admitted. What do you do now?

## CRITICAL THINKING ACTIVITY

Before deciding how you will answer the question, consider the following:

- Teresa's health is improving, but she has a very long way to go before she has a full recovery, which is expected.

- Teresa's parents, while well educated, retain many cultural ideas regarding communication, the role of the family in major decisions, and fears concerning death. They DO NOT WANT HER TOLD.

- Teresa's parents are important allies in her care. They were the only ones who could calm her down when she became agitated or restless. Telling Teresa against their wishes could bring serious long-term negative consequences to Teresa's ability to recover if they refused to help in the future.

You remember previous discussions with the nursing staff. Some of the staff believe her parents are right. Teresa's husband is dead. Telling her now or in the future will not change that. You begin to wonder if it is not your cultural bias that she should be told.

**Decide how you will answer Teresa's question, "Where is my husband?" Write a script for the conversation that follows Teresa's question.** Write the entire script—until the conversation has reached a conclusion. In the dialogue, be sure to bring out all the issues which brought you to answer the question the way you did.

Also describe how the parents reacted—add their facial expressions, tone of voice, and mannerisms. Do the same for yourself and Teresa. Make the conversation come alive with your script.

Consider comparing notes with others in your class who took a different view point.

# Who Decides Who Talks?

A hospice nurse working in an inpatient unit for the terminally ill is stopped outside the door of a patient's room by the patient's mother. The mother is also a nurse from another part of the country. The mother is pleasant and agreeable most of the time, except today. She tells her daughter's nurse that she wants to make sure that no one talks to her about her death and dying process. The nurse is caught cold in her tracks. The woman's daughter is within days of death. The patient is no longer able to eat. Her cardiomyopathy (from drug abuse) has progressed to the point that she is not even able to raise her hands above her head to brush her beautiful blonde hair. This is something she used to love to do.

The nurse listens patiently to the patient's mother. She encourages the mother to verbalize her feelings of frustration, grief, and loss. The mother tells the nurse "how good" her daughter was when she was little. She further recalls that her daughter had always had "bad luck" with friends. And it was these friends who recently planted cocaine in her daughter's room that led to her most recent prison stay. She has been released to hospice pending her death.

After a considerable amount of time, the nurse pauses and tells the mother gently and supportively that her daughter is an adult and still mentally competent, so she is entitled to make her own decisions. The nurse cannot honor her request to refrain from discussing death. This is an essential part of hospice; her daughter also has a right to grieve for all of her losses now, and there is no way to facilitate that without bringing it up.

With that, the mother bursts into tears of both sorrow and rage. She adamantly tells the nurse that she will not allow death to be brought up! She will do "whatever it takes" to stop the nurse from bringing it up.

## CRITICAL THINKING ACTIVITY

It is an ethical imperative that death be openly discussed with all patients, especially those who are dying. **What is to be done now? And by whom?**

Reflect on this situation for awhile. Put yourself in the place of the patient, the mother, and the nurse. How does it feel to be in each person's "shoes?" What is it like to be demanding something you feel so strongly about—the wish to not have death discussed—and to be a nurse and know that what you are asking is NOT ethical by your own code? What does this say about the relationship of the mother and the daughter? What are the implications for the nurse? She may proceed and discuss death with the daughter, but it is the MOTHER who will remain around for awhile and can cause considerable suffering for the nurse. How can that be handled?

**Write a script for the mother, the nurse, and the patient, detailing their conversation about death.** It may or may not be one conversation. Your script should reflect your understanding of the nursing imperatives in this situation, ethics and legal guidelines as they apply, and skill in psychosocial care.

# H I N T S H I N T S H I N T S H I N T S H I N T S

You may want to interview some hospice nurses and ask them what they would do. They have surely been in a similar situation many times!

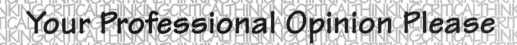

# Your Professional Opinion Please

You are a nurse practitioner in private practice. A new client comes in for a physical. During the course of the examination, she requests the test to see if she has the breast cancer gene. She is willing to pay for the test herself. But she insists on using another name for the test because she does not want a positive test result on her medical record. The client is very concerned about her ability to get insurance in the future if she changes her job. She believes that a positive test result will be considered a "pre-existing" condition and she will be denied medical insurance as a result.

The client has vague reasons for wanting to have the test but is adamant about doing it. As the nurse practitioner, you are a client advocate. But the client has now told you she wants to use an alias for the test. This complicates the matter for you. As a professional, you wonder what you should do now. If you refer her for the test knowing she is going to use an alias, there is a risk of a fraud charge if you are found out, which is unlikely. What will you do with the test results? Put them in her regular file with her real name? Throw your copy of the test results out so there is no evidence that you know what the results are? What will you do if the results come back positive and you need to follow up on them?

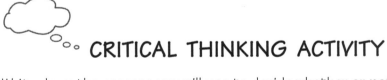 CRITICAL THINKING ACTIVITY

Write down the process you will use to decide whether **or not** you will refer this client for the screening test for the breast cancer gene. Be very specific in listing the ethical principles that guide your decision-making.

If you decide to refer her for the test using an alias, what you will do with the medical records? If you decide not to refer her, what will you do as her advocate for better health? Be specific.

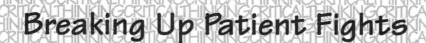

# Breaking Up Patient Fights

You are caring for a patient with a life-threatening condition. While you are changing a central line dressing on the patient, his son comes in to visit. You are glad to see the son here because you heard in report that the father and son have not spoken in over 10 years because of a family argument. Because the patient's condition is serious and he is not expected to live, you are happy that they are making amends before the patient's death.

Just as you begin the dressing change, at a point where you cannot stop, the son begins to pour his heart out his father. The son begins by telling his father how sorry he is for taking the previous argument personally and not staying in contact through the years. But he is glad they have time to spend together now. You feel awkward listening to this deeply personal exchange. You are also deeply touched by the son's loving words.

Just as you finish up the dressing change, the patient begins his replies to the son. In the most angry and hurtful voice imaginable, the father responds with a litany of criticisms and complaints about the son's behavior in the last few years. (The patient is the one who severed relations with the rest of the family; all members had previously shared that with the staff). You cannot believe what you are hearing! You wonder what to do.

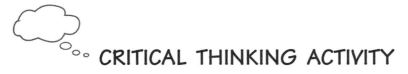

## CRITICAL THINKING ACTIVITY

What will you do next?

You have a few choices. Do you intervene to get the patient to stop talking? Do you let the conversation reach a natural end? Do you help the son stand up to his father? Do you get additional support from other workers, such as a social worker or nursing colleague?

Identify the ethical principles you will use to guide your decision-making process. Be sure to identify the ethical guidelines that pertain to interventions you make on behalf of the client or the son. They may be different.

Finally, ask yourself if the fact that the patient is dying influences your decision, and include that answer in your paper.

# Legal Customers Only Please

Description: Many states have or are considering banning medical care for noncitizens. The situation is dire in some cases. Publicly funded medical facilities have taken patients out of a bed and denied them care when it was learned that the patient was not a citizen. In some cases, the patient was wheeled out instead of walking because he was too sick to walk.

Nurses are often the individuals who have to inform patients that they are being denied or will be denied care for a reason other than medical necessity. There are significant ethical issues raised by these institutional policies. Nurses would do well to consider what their reaction would be to turning an admitted patient away who divulged he was not a citizen.

Put yourself in the place of a staff nurse doing an admission to the surgical unit. You are admitting a patient for a hysterectomy, being done for cervical cancer. You begin talking to the patient and her family during the routine history and physical. In the course of talking to the patient, she tells you that the reason she doesn't work is that she is not a legal citizen and has no right to work. Your heart sinks. Your facility has a mandatory reporting policy when a staff member knows a patient is not a legal citizen. Now what?

You excuse yourself from the room to collect your thoughts. You want to assess the situation and consider your alternatives. The first option that comes to mind is to say nothing. After all who could find out? After a moment or two you realize this patient could tell anyone and let them know she told you, too. You decide you have to notify your supervisor.

 CRITICAL THINKING ACTIVITY

Prepare a short script, less than 5 minutes in length, which will:

1. Let the patient know you are going to report her noncitizenship status

2. Consider what she will say in response to this news

3. What you will tell your supervisor

4. What you will tell the surgeon

Initiate any security measures you need for personal safety. What needs to be done to ensure that the patient or her family will not retaliate against you? Prepare your personal safety plan, and be prepared to share that, too.

# One Last Snowfall

A patient whose condition is deteriorating comes to the medical floor. This patient has a chronic degenerating illness that is in the final stages. On her orders, the physician has noted "no CPR." You know her pretty well because she has had many hospitalizations in the last year. Your intuition tells you that she will not make it out of the hospital this time.

During the admission assessment, the patient tells you she would like to feed the ducks in the hospital water ponds one last time. This could very well be her last request. You are moved by the gentleness of this request. She has no family; the nurses have become her surrogate grievers and well wishers.

It's close to your break time, and you decide you will take her out to feed the ducks during your break. She is getting weaker by the moment and you worry that she will be completely worn out by this energy expenditure. However, the patient's dying wish seems to clearly take precedence in determining your nursing action.

You take her out to feed the ducks and bring her back to her room, where she dies a few hours later. You chart your nursing care plan, actions, and evaluation of the patient's response to your interventions.

The next day your manager calls you at home and asks you to come to the hospital before your shift to talk about an urgent matter. You meet your manager and find that you are being reprimanded for "endangering patient safety" by taking this patient out to the water ponds the day before!

At first you don't know what to make of this. You are shocked that this counseling report has such statements as the "patient could have died while being outside" and "the nurse used poor judgment in granting the patient's inappropriate request." The manager gives you the shift off and demands that you sign the counseling form. You agree to sign it once you have provided a rebuttal of the situation. You go home to prepare your response.

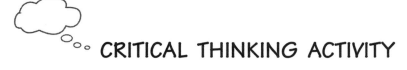 CRITICAL THINKING ACTIVITY

Prepare a written response to this counseling form. Use your knowledge of legal, ethical, and professional guidelines to prepare your answer. Be clear in your thinking about why this act of caring was THE only appropriate action under the circumstances.

# H I N T S HINTS H I N T S HINTS H I N T S

Remember you are fighting for your job. A job you need. So it may not serve your long-term employment interests to be too bold in your comments

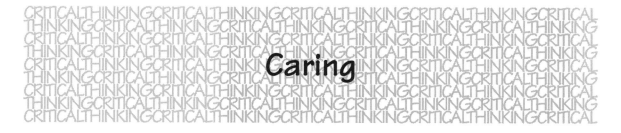

# Caring

There is a great deal of professional discussion and research on the topic of caring and nursing. It has been an immensely important topic to nursing, since the beginning of the profession.

Florence Nightingale wrote about caring indirectly:

All hurry and bustle is peculiarly painful to the sick . . . Always sit down when a sick person is talking to you, show no signs of hurry, give complete attention and full consideration if your advice is wanted . . . Always sit within the patient's view, so that when you speak to him he has not painfully to turn his head round in order to look at you . . . Never speak to an invalid from behind, nor from the door, nor from any distance . . . (*Notes on Nursing*, p. 28).

Madeline Leininger developed the theory of Culture Care. She defined care as: . . . "the essence of nursing and the dominant and unifying domain of nursing."

Jean Watson developed her theory of "Human Caring." Acknowledging Nightingale's legacy of caring, Ms. Watson wrote:

Caring writing today shares a century old national and global agenda with Nightingale. We continue to be informed and inspired by the rich, often hidden, ordinary caring-healing knowing of nursing and women. . . . Ordinary knowing becomes extraordinary when we enter into human caring with a spiritual sense of awe and reverence, with a sense of the fantastic.

Nel Noddings adds to the field of caring with her examination of what it means to care and be cared for. She has presented a theory of moral reasoning based on caring principles. She presents an argument for moral reasoning based on relatedness instead of logic.

 **CRITICAL THINKING ACTIVITY**

Consider these different approaches to caring behaviors. Reflect on your own ideas about the value of caring for others in the nursing sense of the term. Prepare a paper or conduct a discussion on the topic of caring. Address following questions:

Can nurses be forced to care?

Can a demand be made for someone to care?

Can a patient recover from an illness without being "cared for?"

Is there a difference in nursing behaviors that have the underlying principles of: "I care for my patients" versus "I must care for my patients"

What is the difference between caring and acting?

# REFERENCES

Nodding, N. (1984) Caring a Feminine Approach to Ethics and Moral Education. Los Angeles, CA: University of California Press.

Leininger, M. (1988) Care: The Essence of Nursing & Health. Detroit, MI: Wayne State University Press.

Watson, J. (1985) Nursing: Human Science & Human Care. Norwalk, CT: Appleton-Century Crofts.

# Disagreeing With Extraordinary Measures

A patient is brought into the emergency room by ambulance. She is clearly in shock with diminished pulses and cool and cyanotic extremities. Her blood pressure is barely palpable, but she is talking. She is complaining of pain. Her condition is deteriorating rapidly. It is clear she will not be conscious for long. The attending physician has begun to order a series of tests in order to determine the exact nature of the patient's condition. In the meantime, the physician has requested that the family stay in the waiting room until the tests are completed.

In your opinion, the patient will die before the radiology and lab tests are completed on a stat basis. You feel strongly that the patient should be kept with her family during the last moments of her life. You are the only who seems to notice this dilemma. You wait a while to see if your intuition directs your next course of action.

You notice the patient is quieting down. She has gotten a small amount of morphine sulfate for her pain, but she is quieter than you suspect she should be with the narcotic dose given to her. Her vitals are unchanged; they are still poor. You decide to ask the doctor if the family can come in now. He declines, saying that they will just get in the way of the portable x-ray machine and the technicians coming to draw the blood samples.

 CRITICAL THINKING ACTIVITY

**What will you do next?** Consider your ethical obligations to the patient and family in this dire circumstance. There is no question that this patient is dying before your eyes. The lab and other tests will simply confirm the obvious. So now your job turns to preparing the patient and family for goodbyes. But this will be extremely difficult to do because you are not receiving any support for your gentle suggestions of putting aside the convenience of health care workers in order to promote end-of-life resolution. This is typical of this emergency room staff. Dying patients are often left alone. It is as if the patients who will not survive get a different level of care than those who are expected to live.

Write a script **detailing** what you will do next and with whom you will communicate. Will you go to the waiting room and get the family? If so, what will you tell them? Will you try to reason with the emergency department doctor?

How much time will you spend on actions with an uncertain outcome? It may be that you just let the situation evolve on its own. After all, the family knew the patient was in serious condition—they called the emergency medical services center for help. Not all situations need intervention—is this an example of a situation without a solution?

Share your action plan with members of your group. Consider presenting a role play that considers all of the best solutions from your group.

# CHAPTER

# 5

# ADVANCED CRITICAL THINKING ACTIVITIES

# What's Really Wrong Here?

A nursing student accompanied a hospice nurse on her usual daily home care visits. The staff nurse was not happy to have a student "tagging along" but agreed to have her for 1 day only. One of the more routine visits was to Mrs. R., who was dying of end-stage heart disease. She had had several episodes of uncompensated congestive heart failure in the last several months, for which she was hospitalized. During her last hospitalization, she was told that her heart was failing and that nothing more could be done for her. She took this news "in stride" and asked to go home to die.

Mrs. R. had a very attentive family. One of her children and usually several of her grandchildren were always at her side. On this day the student volunteered to take her vital signs, although she was nervous about giving care in someone's home and having so many people watching her. The hospice nurse went in the other room to check on Mrs. R's medication supplies. The student placed the cuff on Mrs. R's arm and remembered she had forgotten her stethoscope in the car. She dashed out to get it and took the blood pressure without delay when she returned. When she removed the cuff, the family members in the room noticed that the cuff had left an imprint on Mrs. R's arm. They became very alarmed at this and called the hospice nurse back into the room. They demanded an explanation of what had happened to cause such an alteration in the skin.

The hospice nurse simply said that the student had made a mistake and left the cuff on too long. The family told the nurse that the student had left the cuff on while she went to her car. Once again, the hospice nurse took an opportunity to further admonish the student to be more thoughtful of patient comfort. Mrs. R never said a word during this entire episode and was alert to everything that happened.

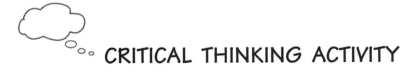

## CRITICAL THINKING ACTIVITY

Review this scenario several times. Diagram or cluster the events as they happened. **Determine what damage to Mrs. R, if any, was created by the cuff; be specific in describing the signs and symptoms you would use to assess potential damage. Determine what could have been done differently.** What could the student have done differently? Should the student have spoken up in her defense? Was this a missed opportunity for family teaching by the hospice nurse?

**Determine what should be done now.** Should an incident report be filled out? If so, what would you say on the report?

**Produce a script of the exchange between the hospice nurse and the student that should take place after the incident. What needs to be said?**

# Culture and Advance Directives

Advance directives are a patient's right in the United States. All patients have the right to specify the extent to which life-saving procedures will be used to prolong their lives. However, we live in a multicultural society, and advance directives are a product of white upper class legislators. These legislators have good intentions and the best interest of all Americans at heart, but do all Americans, with their various cultural backgrounds, support the idea of advance directives? How about various religious and spiritual traditions? Do advance directives make sense through the "lens" of all religions?

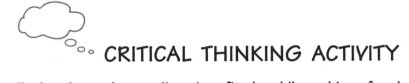 CRITICAL THINKING ACTIVITY

**Explore how advance directives fit the philosophies of various groups of people.** Consider your community and its ethnic and religious diversity. Identify the larger subgroups of people in your community, and critique the use of advance directives within those groups.

Consider citizens of Asian, European, Mexican, South American, and African descent. How does culture play a role in making an advance directive?

Consider citizens of Buddhist, Catholic, Jewish, Moslem, and indigenous religious traditions. How does spiritual faith affect the individual's "need" for an advance directive?

**Write a script for one religion and one subculture of your community in which you, the nurse, describe an advance directive.** What concerns would someone from that background have? Consider what questions the other person in the conversation might have.

Be prepared to share these scripts and develop a resource folder for your class.

# Medication Error: Advanced Chapter

Description: As a nurse you give a patient the wrong medication. The patient does not appear immediately affected by the medication. You are sitting down to write the incident report. One of the items to be filled in on the report asks for you to describe the nursing interventions you will use to assess any potential negative affects that the wrong medication may have on the patient. You called the physician and told him. He was in surgery, and the nurse said to call him if there are ". . . any problems". The pharmacists are in a meeting and are only available for "emergencies." You are pretty sure this is not an emergency. Your job is to complete the incident report and write a plan for the staff to follow in which you describe what side effects to look for in this patient. The first part of the plan will include your assessment of the seriousness of this medication error.

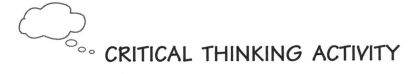

## CRITICAL THINKING ACTIVITY

Describe how you decided this medication error was not serious. What steps did you follow to assess this? What additional information did you gather to support your conclusion that it was not serious? What is your legal liability, and what is the liability of the agency you work in? Share your explanation with one other person, before sharing this in class.

# Regulations on Top of Regulations

Many agencies regulate nursing education and nursing practice. Often it is difficult to keep them all straight and understand the relationship of each one to the others. However, it is very important to know which agencies are regulating which activities and to be able to identify common issues among them. Agencies such as your State Board of Nursing, the American Nurses Association, The Joint Commission on Accreditation of Healthcare Organizations, the National League for Nursing, the American Association of Colleges of Nursing, the Health Care Financing Administration, and various specialty organizations have their own sets of guidelines.

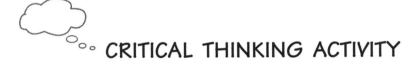

## CRITICAL THINKING ACTIVITY

**Explore how these guidelines fit together by focusing on a few common nursing functions.**

Select one specific component of nursing care—a common nursing issue such as medication administration, making staff assignments, obtaining consents for procedures, or nursing care planning.

**Produce a diagram or other illustration showing the interrelationships, duplication, and gaps in the guidelines of all the agencies that regulate nursing education, nursing practice, and reimbursement for nursing services.** Do not produce a narrative paper!

## HINTSHINTSHINTSHINTSHINTS

You may want to write an article for a local newspaper or a nursing journal with your findings.

# Reasoned Judgment

As the field of critical thinking has developed since the 1950s, so has the definition of critical thinking. Beginning with a definition that reflected a concern for rules of arguments and logic, critical thinking has now evolved into a field that emphasizes reasoned judgment. This means that when a nurse makes a decision about what to do in a given situation, he or she is making that decision based on facts, the context in which the decision is being made, and any related laws and policies. Although people may refer to the decision as the nurse's opinion, it is NOT a subjective personal value statement. In fact, the nurse's decision is like that of a judge in a court room. The decision is one that reflects knowledge and understanding, not personal bias.

The next series of activities is the culminating work of this text. Your work should reflect your understanding of the basic rules of argument that you received in nursing prerequisite courses and the principles you have learned in nursing school. As you work through each activity, it is important that you see yourself as a judge of the facts, of what is relevant to the issue, and of what the priorities are. You may want to make notes to yourself all along the path of decision-making. This will allow you to go back and question yourself regarding your underlying assumptions, facts, and related information.

Be cautioned! Making a sound judgment takes time and thought. It is a skill and an art. Knowledge in nursing is a given, as is your desire for truth, an understanding of the context in which the decision is being made, and the available resources. The ability to make sound judgments is an essential skill for nurses in the 21st century!

# Who Gets A Transplant?

A 20-year-old man comes into the emergency department in critical condition. He recently ingested a large number of barbiturates in an attempt to kill himself. He was not found until a significant amount of time had gone by, and he is suffering from multiple organ failure. However, there is a chance he could survive with a liver transplant. This patient has been out of work for a while because of depression, so he has no insurance. It will be necessary to apply for Medicaid or state-funded health care coverage for him.

His doctor calls you at the local organ procurement alliance and asks for the man to be placed at the top of the list for liver transplants—the patient will surely die within the next couple of days without a transplant. As the transplant coordinator, you are responsible for notifying the Allocation Committee about such emergencies. With your prior knowledge about who is on the waiting list, you realize this will place the patient above other people who have been waiting for a longer period of time and who have liver failure from various diseases—not self-induced conditions.

You feel that there are ethical and practical issues in this situation. For example, assuming this patient gets a liver, what are the chances he will try to take his life again—thereby wasting that organ? There are so few organs available for transplant that this seems to you to be an unacceptable option. In addition, you wonder what the ethical issues are regarding giving preference to someone who put themselves in a position of needing an organ transplant versus someone needing a transplant who had no control over his or her disease.

## CRITICAL THINKING ACTIVITY

**If a patient causes his liver failure, should he be allowed to be placed at the top of the organ recipient list?**

Write a memo to the Allocation Committee describing your recommendations about placing this man on the top of the transplant recipient list. Detail the issues as you see them, and make a recommendation about his location on the list. You must use reasoned judgment to complete this activity. Use laws, ethical guidelines, and nursing knowledge to guide you in writing the memo. Be clear about your sources. Be able to identify the sources of your comments in class. Compare your recommendations with those of others in the class.

# Who Pays for What?

You are a case manager for a workers' compensation insurance company. The supervisor of the claims department has asked you to decide a sticky issue in a case. The claimant received a back injury at work after a minor fall. Initially he received a medical workup and treatment. This included time off from work, medication, and physical therapy, and ultimately he was returned to a light duty assignment. After several weeks of care, he did not improve. His physician recommended admission to the hospital for close observation and further testing.

After the first few tests were done, a large malignant tumor was found to be pressing on his spinal cord and was thought to be the source of his symptoms from the beginning. The claims supervisor is furious that no one had discovered this tumor before the insurance company had paid out so much money in medical care and time off from work. He wants you to "find a way" to deny this claim. Specifically, he wants you to write a report that details the reasons why the whole claim should be thrown out, releasing the company from responsibility for the most recent hospitalization.

He is not asking you to practice medicine without a license. He is asking you to use your nursing knowledge to describe in plain English, for the claims review committee and the employer (who ultimately pays the claim through the insurance company), why this injury was not work related. Once it is established that the claimant's symptoms were related to the cancer and not the fall he sustained at work, the supervisor will be "off the hook" for this very large claim.

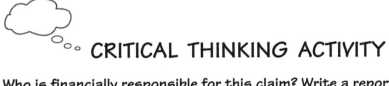

## CRITICAL THINKING ACTIVITY

**Who is financially responsible for this claim? Write a report detailing your recommendations about who has the financial responsibility for this claim.** Consider all sides of the issue. Use your sense of fairness and fiscal responsibility to get you started. Think of short- and long-term consequences for every possible solution you identify. Look at the situation from the claimant's perspective, the employer's perspective, and the insurance carrier's perspective. How much financial responsibility should each party assume? Describe your thoughts in your report.

# Stereotyping in Charting

You are the preceptor for a newly hired nurse. The new nurse has several years of experience in the area and has been an easy person to orient to the policies and procedures of your unit. Consistently you have seen her demonstrate a caring and knowledgeable approach to patients and their families. She has worked well with minimal supervision. Until today, you have not seen any reason to consider her anything other than a nice addition to the staff.

Upon review of her charting—during a routine spot check that is periodically required of you throughout the preceptorship—you notice an inappropriate comment on a discharge note. The new nurse has written discharge instructions for a patient who is going home from the hospital post–open reduction internal fixation of a left hip fracture. The new nurse has indicated that she taught the patient how to do a non–weight-bearing transfer between the bed and chair. The patient returned the demonstration with no difficulty and clearly understands her restrictions at home. All of this is documented according to policy in the nursing notes. However, at the end of the record the nurse makes the comment that "She is a credit to her race!" The patient is a woman of color, and the nurse is of European mixed descent, like so many other "Americans." The patient has not seen this notation because you needed to spot check this charting before the nurse had the patient sign it. Everything is complete, except for the patient's confirming receipt of instructions signature.

 CRITICAL THINKING ACTIVITY

**What should you do?** What are your feelings regarding this remark? Should it stay? Is it inappropriate to have the nurse redo this discharge plan? Is that altering a part of the chart after the fact? Is there an issue of cultural bias that reflects on this nurse to the extent that you wonder whether she is an appropriate employee? Is there an issue of discrimination, poor wording, or racism?

**Write a script of the exchange between yourself (the preceptor) and the nurse who made the comment.** What are the relevant issues? What issues take priority over others? Should the record be changed? Plan to act your script out in class.

# What Are the Obstacles?

Every nursing student learns the basics of authentic communication, methods for resolving difficult health- and illness-related problems, and a method of describing measurable actions and goals (the nursing care plan). Yet when those same nursing students go into health care facilities, they often find less than optimal use of interviewing techniques, acceptance of patients just as they are, and work on issues "where you find them," like dealing with an alcoholic patient from his own perspective, rather than imposing the nurses' own value judgments on their patients' behavior.

The reasons for this inability to fully integrate theoretical knowledge with practical knowledge are complex and deep in our systems of interpersonal interaction, leadership models, values, and concerns about being accepted as a member of the dominant group, among other reasons. The problem is so pervasive that many students assume they will disregard much of what they learn in school and do things the way the staff does them.

Sometimes this is a conscious decision, perhaps based on personal values, and sometimes it may come as a result of not seeing another way. Perhaps it is from not being able to fully integrate the principles taught in nursing school with the principles practiced on the job, regardless of the health care setting, for other reasons.

However, it doesn't have to be this way . . .

## CRITICAL THINKING ACTIVITY

Divide your class into small groups, or self-select small discussion groups. **Explore the question: What prevents student nurses from carrying the values they have learned in nursing school directly to the job?**

You may come up with a number of obvious answers at first, including time constraints, too many patients, no one wants to, etc. Keep discussing the topic until you hear your group getting to the deeper causes of this inability to realize the full potential of nursing.

**Once you have gotten to some of the underlying issues, draw a diagram that shows the key points and describes the interrelationship of these points and any smaller points.** Plan to share your results with the larger class. Draw your diagram on an

$8\frac{1}{2}$" × 11" sheet of paper so you can turn it into an overhead transparency for ease in presenting it to the class.

**Once your class has shared their results, note the similarities and differences. Define one strategy to ensure that members of your class will carry one value, which they learned in nursing school, forward into practice.**

Identify a method of evaluating your progress with this goal.

# "New Age" Informed Consent

You are planning an inservice on alternative therapies for your nursing staff. Your purpose is to acquaint the nurses in your facility with many local alternative therapists and give them the experience of seeing various therapies that patients use in addition to their traditional medical care. In order to make this fun and useful, several alternative healers will be asking for volunteers from those attending and will demonstrate their techniques. You are very excited about this innovative and much-needed program. You have a reiki master, an expert in aromotherapy, another in music therapy, and one of the most popular alternative healers in the area, a crystal healer.

Just before the inservice starts, the crystal healer comes up to you and tells you that she wants to put certain crystals out in the room, in order to "change the energy." She goes on to say that it isn't necessary for the participants to be aware of what she is doing. This can be done easily by simply placing the crystals and stones at various locations in the room. "They won't even know I am doing anything to them," she tells you.

At first you have no objection. However, as nurses start to arrive and it gets closer to the time to introduce the speakers, you begin to wonder if you are violating principals of informed consent. You are wondering if crystal healing is any different than surgery or other traditional therapy. You ask yourself: Is it legal or ethical to have these crystals lying around the room without the participants knowing that they are being "treated?"

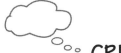 CRITICAL THINKING ACTIVITY

**Answer the question: Is alternative therapy subject to the same laws as traditional medical therapy?** Does your belief as to whether or not crystal healing works influence your decision?

**Prepare a script between you and the healer.** You may want to work in pairs for this activity. Be as comprehensive as you need to be in your script. Make sure that you have resolved the problem for this occasion and future occasions. Writing a policy may be helpful to clarify the entire issue of alternative therapies and informed consent.

# How Has Education Changed?

In his book, *Generation X Goes to College: An Eye-Opening Account of Teaching in Post Modern America*, Peter Sacks describes his reaction to changing professions from journalism to college teaching. Among his comments about college students and instructors, he makes the following observations:

> Pandering to student opinions was the norm at his college.
>
> Many students expected an A or B without working for it; students felt "entitled" to an A or B.
>
> Students told him, through the faculty evaluation process, that they expected a good grade and would give him a poor evaluation if they didn't get one.
>
> Students were comfortable having faculty spoon feed them information for tests because the students knew the faculty needed to have good evaluations in order to get tenure and be successful at the college.
>
> Instructors must keep the students happy and have good evaluations so they "dumb down" the curriculum to ensure this will happen.
>
> He felt amazement when his students felt their opinions were equal to his, even without information on the subject matter.

 CRITICAL THINKING ACTIVITY

**Write down your immediate reactions to Mr. Sacks's analysis of college students and instructors.** Don't worry about the form or grammar, focus on your feelings.

Now sit quietly for 20 minutes and reflect on your college education until now. Do you see any correlation of the author's ideas and your personal experience? If so describe it, giving examples.

**Prepare a paper discussing the implications of the "dumbing down" of curriculum in colleges.** How is nursing different from other majors? Given that you can take the NCLEX and pass with 75 questions—do you think you have enough education to be a competent nurse?

How much do your general education courses support your role as a professional nurse? Skills in writing, speaking, second languages, math, and logic are more important than ever. How well did your education help you master these skills? How much effort did you put into these courses?

**Focus your paper on the underlying assumptions about these courses. Did you feel you should be graded on effort?** Or did you feel you should be graded on knowledge derived from the course that you could demonstrate on papers and tests? Have courage in your analysis! The classes are over; your previous grades will not be changed. This is an opportunity to learn something about your underlying assumptions of your role as a student. Insight into assumptions will help you in your role as a nurse. It will also help you get the most out of the rest of your nursing education.

After reviewing your reaction to Mr. Sacks' comments, write a letter to him. He can be reached at:

Open Court Publishing
315 Fifth Street
PO Box 599
Peru, IL 61354-0599

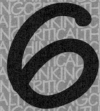
# DEBATE
# TOPICS

# Debate Guidelines

Debates are an excellent method of sharpening thinking skills. They are also a refreshing change from more traditional nursing education methods. Debates are meant to demonstrate both a student's scientific research in a specific area and thinking skills. Debates are NOT a matter of expressing one's personal opinion on a topic. It is not necessary for you to agree on the opinion presented by your team in order to be a convincing debater.

 ## GUIDELINES

Debates follow a variety of guidelines. Use these simple guidelines for the debate topics suggested in this chapter:

1.  Divide your class or group into affirmative and negative teams.

2.  Research the side of the argument your team will be presenting. Be sure to include the most recent and reliable sources of information for your arguments in support of your topic. The reliability of your sources is just as important as the organization of the information and your presentation of same.

3.  Be sure to practice your presentation before the actual classroom presentation. Consider videotaping your presentation for a self-critique.

4.  Time yourself and make adjustments in your presentation as necessary. Timeliness is very important in a debate. You will not be allowed to go over the allotted time for your presentation.

5.  Sequence of presentations:
    Step 1    Affirmative side #1    3 minutes
    Step 2    Negative side #1    3 minutes
    Step 3    Affirmative side #2    3 minutes
    Step 4    Negative side #2    3 minutes
    Step 5    Affirmative rebuttal    3 minutes
    Step 6    Negative rebuttal    3 minutes
    Step 7    Affirmative summary    3 minutes
    Step 8    Negative rebuttal    3 minutes

CRITICALTHINKINGCRITICALTHINKINGCRITICALTHINKINGCRITICALTHINKINGCRITICAL
THINKINGCRITICALTHINKINGCRITICALTHINKINGCRITICALTHINKINGCRITICALTHINKING
CRITICALTHINKINGCRITICALTHINKINGCRITICALTHINKINGCRITICALTHINKINGCRITICAL

# Name Tags

The use of name tags frequently is a legislative issue for health care workers in most states. It may seem like a straight forward issue. All health care workers need to identify themselves to patients and members of the public. However, because of increasing violence against health care workers, there is a risk in doing so. Patients, family, and other visitors to a health care facility can gain access to personal information about employees using the full name read from a name tag.

**Debate Topic:** Name tags should be worn at the discretion of the employee.

# Entry Level Into Practice

The baccalaureate degree (BSN) as the entry level into nursing is fast becoming a reality, both formally through professional association mandates, and informally through hiring practices for many hospitals and health care facilities. Is this subject decided once and for all?

Given the extreme cost control restraints of present health care systems, entry level into practice may need to be reexamined.

**Debate Topic:** Entry level into practice should be a BSN.

# Diseases of Lifestyle and Transplants

Organ donors are a scarce resource in medicine today. The availability of organs is only able to meet a small portion of the need of people with all types of life-threatening diseases. As a result, some prioritizing of potential organ recipients is necessary. One controversial area is the denial of organ transplants to people who are sick from "diseases of lifestyle." Diseases resulting from lifestyle include lung conditions such as emphysema from smoking, cirrhosis of the liver from alcohol abuse, and heart disease from risk factors such as a sedentary lifestyle, a high-fat diet, and the like.

**Debate Topic:** Individuals considered for organ transplant should be only those people with diseases associated with infection, trauma, genetic disposition, or other etiology NOT associated with the patient's voluntary lifestyle prior to the illness.

# Fetal Brain Tissue Transplants

Before the increasing demand for prohibition on abortion and decreasing supply of fetuses, much neurologic research was being done using brain tissue from aborted fetuses. Parkinson's disease is one condition for which there is the possibility of a substantially increased quality of life after fetal brain transplant. However, since the presidential order banning such transplants, research in the area has stagnated.

**Debate Topic:** Fetal tissue should be available for medical research.

# Research on Animals

The suffering of helpless animals is one of the great social concerns in this country and others. A great deal of money is donated to causes that seek to decrease the pain and suffering of animals of all kinds, especially dogs and other animals used in medical research.

Many research studies were abandoned after animal rights activists broke into research labs, stealing research animal subjects. The efforts of many people and animals were wasted as a result of a premature ending to these studies.

Although no one wants to see animals suffer needlessly, humans may very well suffer needlessly because of the zealousness of a few activists.

**Debate Topic:** Animals should be used in approved medical research studies.

# Residents With the Right to Fall

The use of physical restraints is growing more controversial all the time. Many states have banned the use of restraints, citing the rationale that residents of long-term care facilities and other health care agencies should receive the benefit of alternative interventions to protect them from falling.

Another central consideration in the restraint debate is that residents of long-term care facilities are encouraged to view their rooms as they did their homes. Few people are restrained in their own homes. The government sees these individuals, regardless of the decline in their mental capacity, as having significant rights to self-determination. As such, they have the "right to fall."

**Debate Topic:** Patients/residents/clients in extended care facilities with a history of falling must be restrained when their physical and mental capacity jeopardizes their safety.

# Physician-Assisted Suicide

The court system is trying to determine which patients, under which conditions, can request physician-assisted suicide. There are many legal, medical, cultural, financial, political, social, and spiritual implications of physician-assisted suicide. As the terms of legal physician-assisted suicide are worked out, nurses, too, must debate and develop professional standards of nursing care for these patients and their families. Now is the time to be thinking about the issue and considering how you see your role as a nurse affected by legalizing physician-assisted suicide.

**Debate Topic:** Physician-assisted suicide should be legalized using strict medical criteria for patient selection.

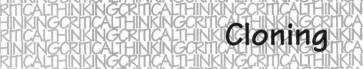

# Cloning

Cloning, or the genetic photocopying of living beings (the first clone reported was Dolly the sheep), is a most controversial issue. The ramifications extend well into the future in ways we cannot even predict. Laws and policies regarding human cloning are in the developmental stage. Currently, human cloning research is illegal. But for how long? Are there benefits to cloning? What are the social, moral, political, and other consequences?

**Debate Topic:** All cloning research should continue in government-sanctioned research studies.

# Care Plan Substitutes

Nursing care plans are inconsistently used. Many staff nurses fail to see their benefit, and some systems of charting make them time consuming and impractical. Others feel that all care should flow from the medical diagnosis only. Nursing experts point to the need for nursing practice to ensure professional stature. The issue is complex and significant.

**Debate Topic:** Care plans should be replaced with a plan of care based on the medical problems of the patient.

# HIV Positive Patients Must Inform Health Care Workers

People with HIV and/or AIDS do not currently have to divulge that fact to health care workers, because of a potential violation of privacy. However, all other patients are expected to be forthright in giving health care workers information about their health histories. Is there a double standard here? Or is the discrimination faced by people with HIV and AIDS so different that special protection is required?

**Debate Topic:** Patients receiving health care of any kind must be required to reveal whether they are HIV positive.

# Equal Access to Health Care is a Right

The working poor are increasingly without health insurance. Very poor people can get some medical care at the expense of the taxpayers. More and more middle class workers will be without health insurance if costs continue to rise and employers are not able to afford the premiums. Many public health concerns can be eliminated or minimized with proper, inexpensive health care, such as immunizations for all children and flu shots on demand for all people. Is it fair that only the poorest, the richest, and those with good enough jobs get health insurance?

# APPENDIX Internet Addresses

Nursing and Critical Thinking:
http://www.cariboo.bc.ca/psd/nursing/faculty/heaslip/nrsct.htm

National Health Skills Standards Project:
http://www.fwl.org.nhcssp/health.htm

The goal of the National Health Care Skill Standard Project is to develop core standards of skills across many health care disciplines in order to improve health care delivery in the United States. Although critical thinking is not specifically mentioned, it is at the heart of many of the standards which require analysis and evaluation of client data. The entire guideline is available at this URL.

Foundation for Critical Thinking
PO Box 7087
Cotati, CA 94931
707-664-2901
Http://www.sonoma.edu/cthink

Has a wide variety of publications available and sponsors critical thinking conferences all over the United States.

Case students for critical thinking which come from educational settings:
http://www.calpress.com/casindex.htm

Critical thinking information and links:
http://www.iupui.edu/it/edschool/x151/ct.htm

Critical thinking; intellectual standards:
http://w3.ag.uiuc.edu/AIM/Discovery/Mind/crthinking.html

Critical Thinking Bibliography:
http://www.montclair.edu/Pages/CRC/Bibliographies/CriticalThinking.html

Critical Thinking and the Popular Media:
http://www.justthink.org/newindex.asp

CRITICALTHINKINGCRITICALTHINKINGCRITICALTHINKINGCRITICALTHINKINGCRITICAL
THINKINGCRITICALTHINKINGCRITICALTHINKINGCRITICALTHINKINGCRITICALTHINKINGCRITICAL
CRITICALTHINKINGCRITICALTHINKINGCRITICALTHINKINGCRITICALTHINKINGCRITICAL
THINKINGCRITICALTHINKINGCRITICALTHINKINGCRITICALTHINKINGCRITICALTHINKING
CRITICALTHINKINGCRITICALTHINKINGCRITICALTHINKINGCRITICALTHINKINGCRITICAL

# INDEX